The Super Easy Keto Vegetarian Cookbook

Simple and Delicious Vegetarian Recipes to Lose Weight Easily on a Keto Diet Plan

Lidia Wong

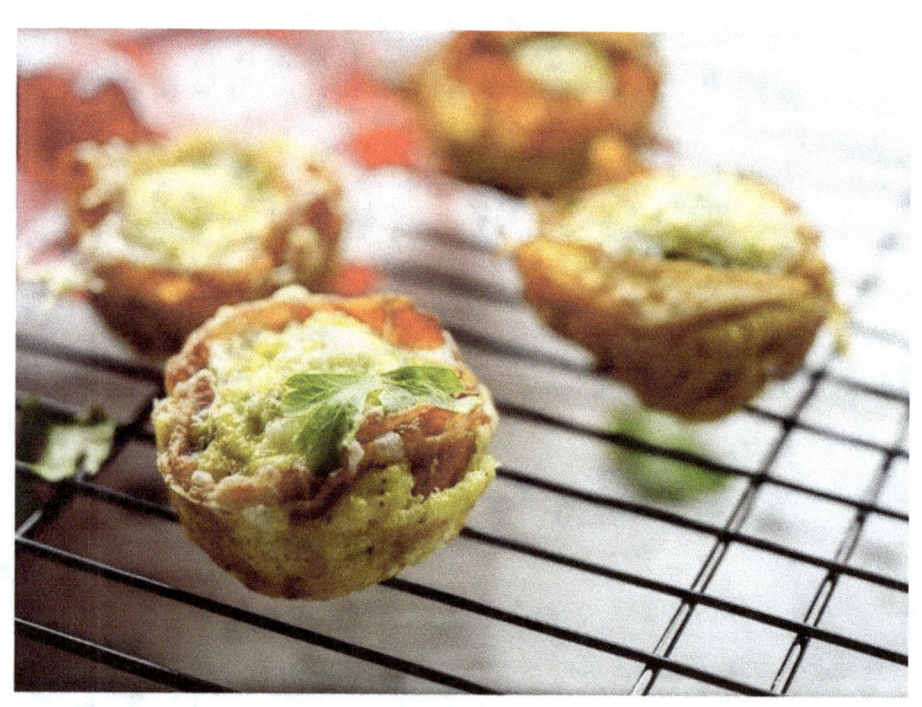

© **Copyright 2021 by Lidia Wong - All rights reserved.**

The content contained within this book may not be reproduced, duplicated or transmitted without direct written permission from the author or the publisher.
Under no circumstances will any blame or legal responsibility be held against the publisher, or author, for any damages, reparation, or monetary loss due to the information contained within this book. Either directly or indirectly.

Legal Notice:
This book is copyright protected. This book is only for personal use. You cannot amend, distribute, sell, use, quote or paraphrase any part, or the content within this book, without the consent of the author or publisher.

Disclaimer Notice:
Please note the information contained within this document is for educational and entertainment purposes only. All effort has been executed to present accurate, up to date, and reliable, complete information. No warranties of any kind are declared or implied. Readers acknowledge that the author is not engaging in the rendering of legal, financial, medical or professional advice. The content within this book has been derived from various sources. Please consult a licensed professional before attempting any techniques outlined in this book.
By reading this document, the reader agrees that under no circumstances is the author responsible for any losses, direct or indirect, which are incurred as a result of the use of information contained within this document, including, but not limited to, — errors, omissions, or inaccuracies.

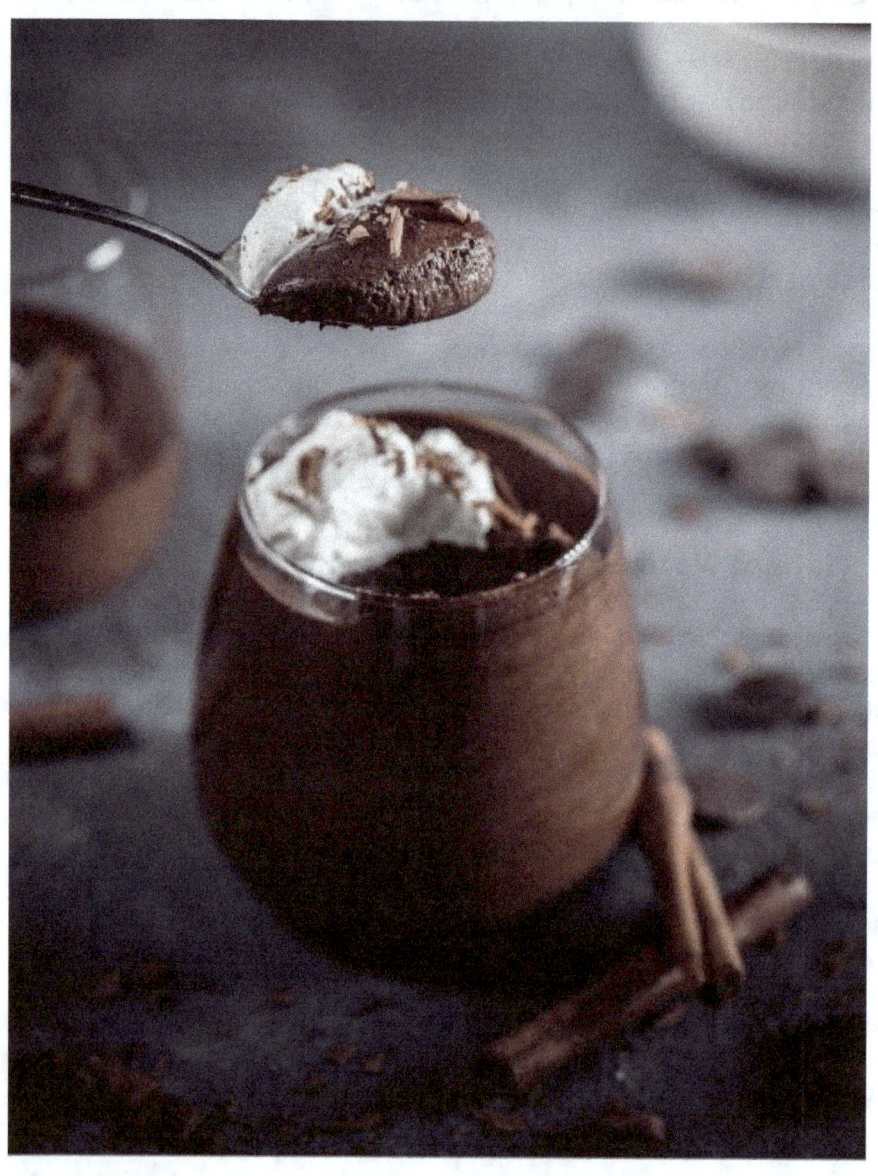

TABLE OF CONTENTS

INTRODUCTION 1

    Almond Cinnamon Smoothie............................. 3

    Mexican Tofu Scramble 5

    Blueberry Soufflé 7

    Celery and Radish Soup 9

    Spinach and Cucumber Salad.........................11

    Spinach and Broccoli Soup 13

    Mushrooms and Chard Soup 15

    Hot Roasted Peppers Cream 17

    Broccoli, Chard and Kale Mix.........................19

    Mashed Cauliflower...21

    Simple Grilled Mushrooms 23

    Braised Seitan with Kelp Noodles 25

    Chili Artichokes...27

    Brussels Sprouts Mix 28

    Tomato Quinoa 30

    Mushrooms and Radishes Mix 32

    Simple Sesame Stir-Fry 34

    Minted Peas...37

Basic Baked Potatoes 39

Orange-Dressed Asparagus............................... 41

Broccoli With Almonds.. 43

Roasted Bell Peppers Soup 45

Cream Of Artichoke Soup 47

Butternut Soup With A Swirl Of Cranberry 49

Mom's Creamy Broccoli and Rice Bake................ 51

Mexican Fideo Soup With Pinto Beans 53

Senegalese Soup.. 55

Greek Potato Salad 57

Quinoa Salad With Black Beans And Tomatoes 59

Balsamic Pearl Onions Bowls 61

Hot Eggplant and Broccoli Spread 62

Coconut Cashew Dip 64

Pomegranate Dip.. 66

Creamy Blackberry Cinnamon Smoothie............. 67

Beans and Spinach Tacos 69

Crispy Kale Chips.. 71

Chinese Soup And Ginger Sauce 73

Eggplant Salad 75

Zucchini & Ricotta Tart 77

Pumpkin Pie Cups (Pressure cooker) 80

Almond Balls 82

Creamy Pineapple Mix 84

Cocoa Muffins 85

Chia and Strawberries Mix 87

Ginger Cream 88

Coconut Chocolate Cake 89

Lime Custard 91

Keto Flax Seed Waffles 92

Cranberries and Avocado Pie 94

Greek Chia Pudding (lacto) 95

Nutty Protein Shake (vegan) 97

Avocado Cucumber Soup 99

NOTE **101**

INTRODUCTION

The keto diet is the shortened term for ketogenic diet and it is essentially a high-fat and low-carb diet that helps you lose weight, thereby bringing various health benefits. This diet drastically restricts your carb intake while increasing your fat intake; this pushes your body to go into a state know as "*ketosis*". We will tackle ketosis in a bit.

The human body uses glucose from carbs to fuel metabolic pathways—meaning various bodily functions like digestion, breathing, etc.. Essentially, anything that needs energy. Even when you are resting, the body needs fuel or energy for you to continue living. If you think about it, when have you ever stopped breathing, or your heart stopped beating, or your liver stopped from cleansing the body, or your kidneys from filtering blood?

Never, unless you're dead, which is the only time in which the body doesn't need energy. In normal circumstances, glucose is the primary pathway when it comes to sourcing the body's energy.

But the body also has another pathway; it can utilize fats to fuel the various bodily processes. And this is what we call "*ketosis*". And the body can only enter ketosis when there is no glucose available, thus the reason for sticking to a low-carb diet is essential in the keto diet. Since no glucose is available, the body is pushed to use fats—it can either come from the food you consume or from your body's fat reserves—the adipose tissue or from the flabby parts of your body. This is how the keto diet helps you lose weight, by burning up all those stored fats that you have and using it to fuel bodily processes.

That said, if for whatever reason you are a vegetarian, following a ketogenic diet can be extremely difficult. A vegetarian diet is largely free of animal products, which means that food tends to be usually high in carbohydrates. Still, with careful planning, it is possible. This Cookbook will provide you with various easy and delicious dishes to help you stick to your ketogenic diet plan while being a vegetarian.

Enjoy!

Almond Cinnamon Smoothie

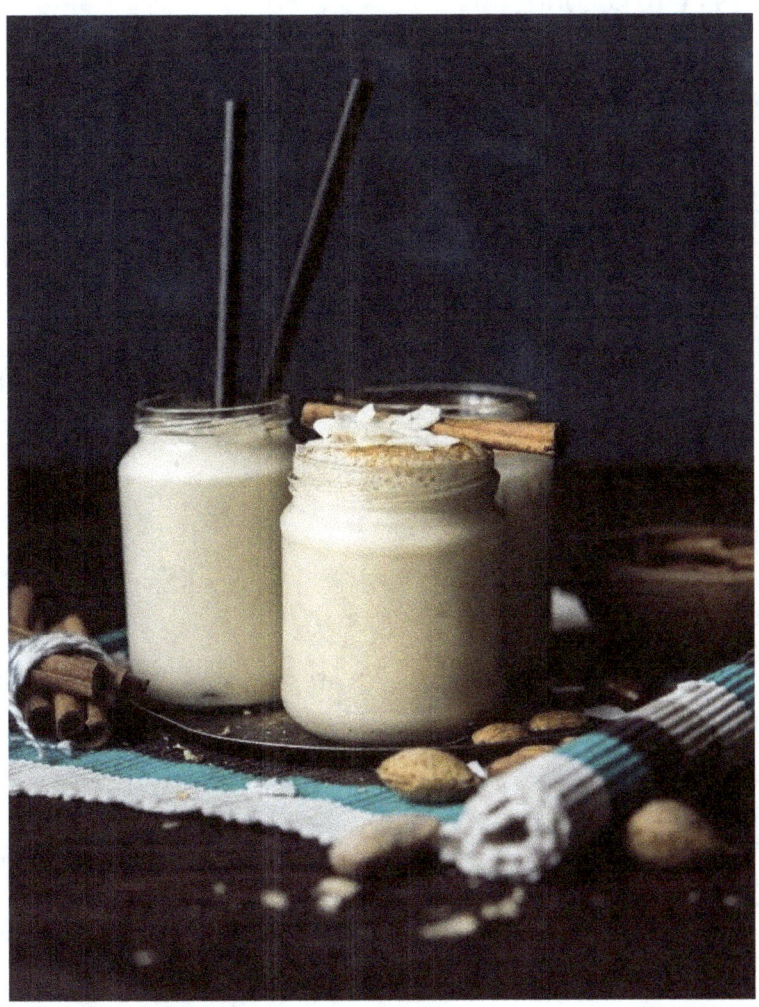

Preparation Time: 10 minutes

Servings: 1

Ingredients:

- ¾ cup almond milk, unsweetened
- ¼ cup coconut oil
- 1 tablespoon vanilla protein powder
- 1 tablespoon almond butter, unsweetened
- 1/8 teaspoon cinnamon

Directions:

1. Add into your blender all the ingredients, blend them until they are nice and smooth.
2. Serve and enjoy!

Nutritional Values (Per Serving):

Calories: 500 Fat: 43 g Carbohydrates: 10 g Sugar: 2 g Protein: 14.6 g Cholesterol: 0 mg

Mexican Tofu Scramble

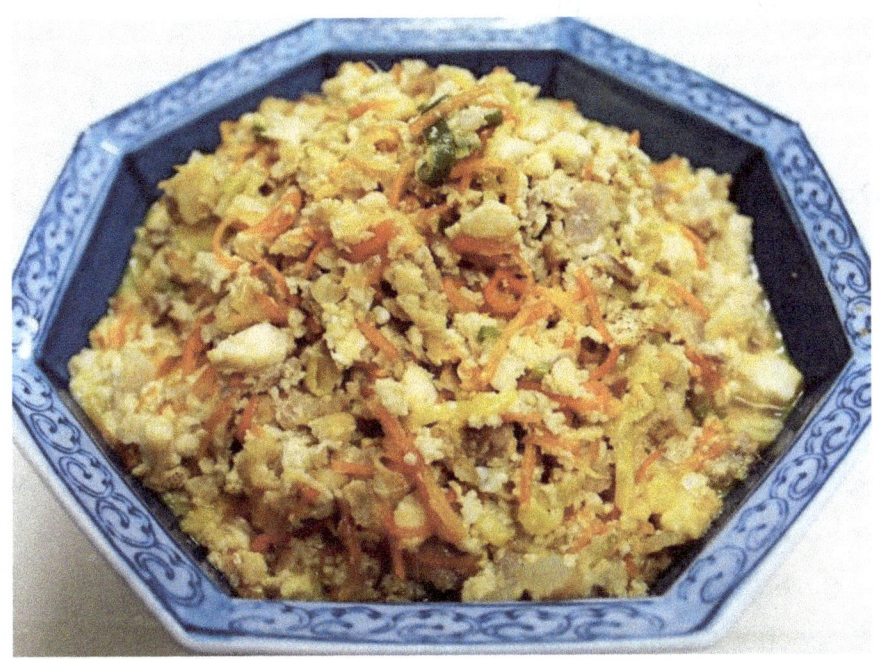

Preparation Time: 34 minutes

Cooking Time: 12 minutes

Serving: 4

Ingredients:

- 2 tbsp olive oil, for frying and crumbled
- 1 green bell pepper, deseeded and finely chopped
- 8 oz extra firm tofu, pressed
- 1 tomato, finely chopped

- 1 tsp Mexican-style chili powder
- 2 tbsp chopped fresh scallions to garnish
- Salt and black pepper to taste
- 3 oz. grated Parmesan cheese

Directions:

1. Heat the olive oil in a medium skillet over medium heat, crumble in the tofu and cook until golden brown, 4 to 6 minutes.
2. Occasionally stir but make sure not to break the tofu into tiny pieces. The goal is to have the tofu looking like scrambled eggs.
3. Stir in the remaining ingredients and cook until the cheese starts melting, 2 minutes.
4. Dish the food and serve warm.

Nutrition:

Calories: 215, Total Fat:16.1 g, Saturated Fat:4.5 g, Total Carbs:7 g, Dietary Fiber: 1g, Sugar:2 g, Protein:12 g, Sodium:402 mg

Blueberry Soufflé

Preparation Time: 15 minutes

Cooking Time: 20 minutes

Serving: 4

Ingredients:

For the blueberry sauce:

- 1 cup frozen blueberries
- 1 tbsp water
- 2 tsp erythritol

For the omelet:

- 4 egg yolks, room temperature
- 1 tsp olive oil
- 3 tbsp erythritol, divided
- 3 egg whites, room temperature
- ½ lemon, zested to garnish

Directions:

For the blueberry sauce:

1. Pour the blueberries, erythritol and water in a small saucepan over medium heat. Cook with occasional stirring until the berries soften and become syrupy, 8 to 10 minutes. Stir in the vanilla, turn the heat off, and set

aside to cool slightly.

For the omelet:

2. Preheat the oven to 350 ºF.
3. In a large bowl, beat the egg yolks and 1 tablespoon of erythritol with an electric whisk until thick and pale. In another bowl, whisk the egg whites at low speed with clean beaters until foamy. Increase the speed, add the remaining erythritol, 1 tablespoon at a time, and whisk until soft peak forms, 3 to 4 minutes. Gently and gradually, fold the egg white mixture into the egg yolk mix.
4. Heat the olive oil in a safe oven non-stick frying pan over low heat. Swirl the pan to spread the oil and pour in the egg mixture; swirl to spread too. Cook for 3 minutes and then, transfer to the oven; bake for 2 to 3 minutes or until golden, puffed, and set.
5. Plate the omelet and spoon the blueberry sauce onto the egg. Use the spoon to spread around. Garnish with lemon zest.
6. Serve immediately with tea or coffee.

Nutrition:

Calories:478, Total Fat: 46.8g, Saturated Fat:27.3 g, Total Carbs: 8 g, Dietary Fiber: 4g, Sugar: 1g, Protein: 11g, Sodium: 257mg

Celery and Radish Soup

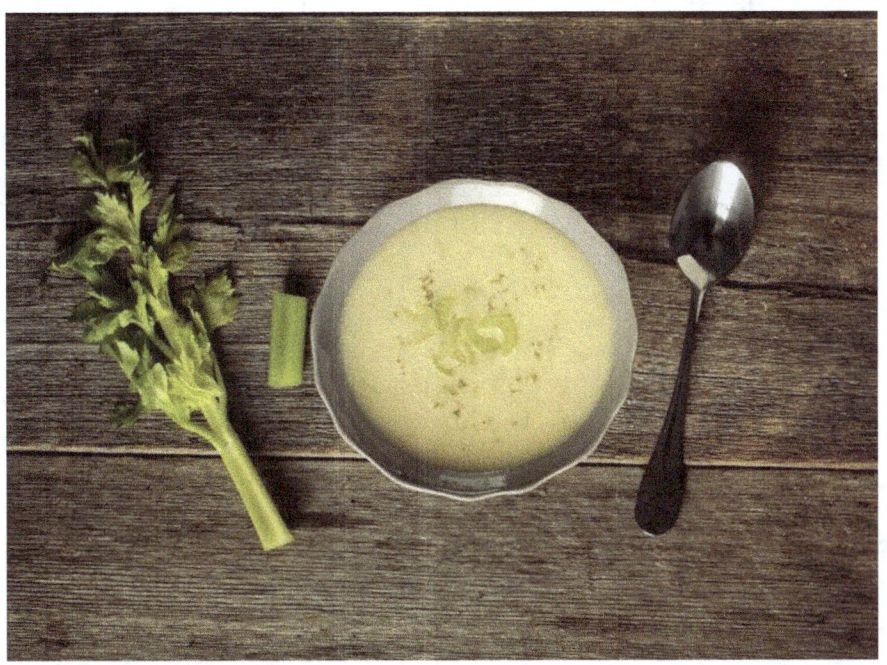

Preparation time: 10 minutes

Cooking time: 20 minutes

Servings: 4

Ingredients:

- ½ pound radishes, cut into quarters
- 2 tablespoons olive oil
- 2 celery stalks, chopped

- 1 teaspoon fennel seeds, crushed
- 4 scallions, chopped
- 1 teaspoon coriander, dried
- 6 cups vegetable stock
- Salt and black pepper to the taste
- 6 garlic cloves, minced
- 1 tablespoon chives, chopped

Directions:

1. Heat up a pot with the oil over medium heat, add the celery, scallions and the garlic and sauté for 5 minutes.
2. Add the radishes and the other ingredients, bring to a boil, cover and simmer for 15 minutes.
3. Divide into soup bowls and serve.

Nutrition:

calories 120, fat 2, fiber 1, carbs 3, protein 10

Spinach and Cucumber Salad

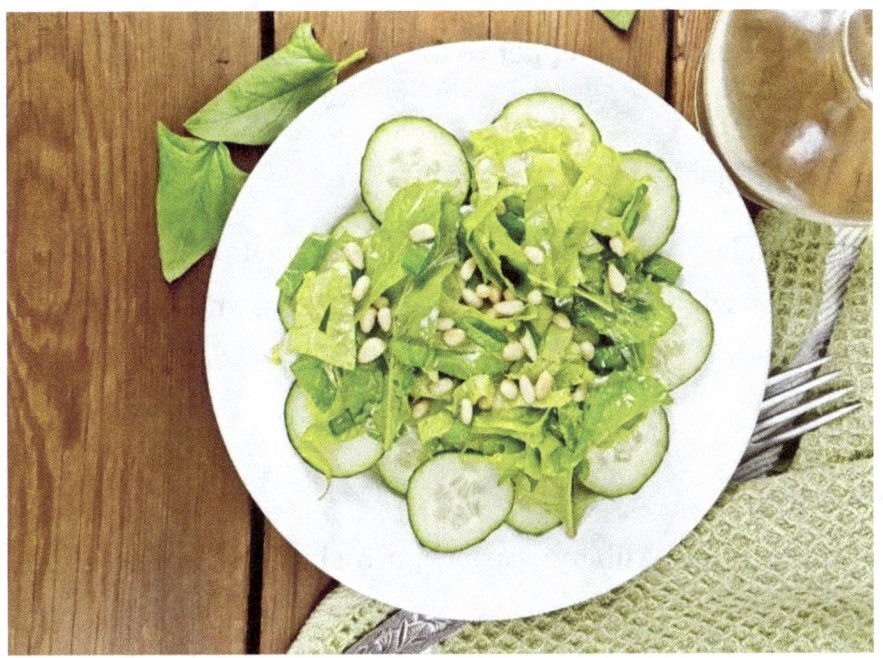

Preparation time: 5 minutes

Cooking time: 0 minutes

Servings: 4

Ingredients:

- 1 pound cucumber, sliced
- 1 tablespoon chili powder
- 2 cups baby spinach

- ¼ cup cilantro, chopped
- 2 tablespoons olive oil
- 2 tablespoons lemon juice
- Salt and black pepper to the taste

Directions:

1. In a large salad bowl, combine the cucumber with the spinach and the other ingredients, toss and serve for lunch.

Nutrition:

calories 140, fat 4, fiber 2, carbs 4, protein 5

Spinach and Broccoli Soup

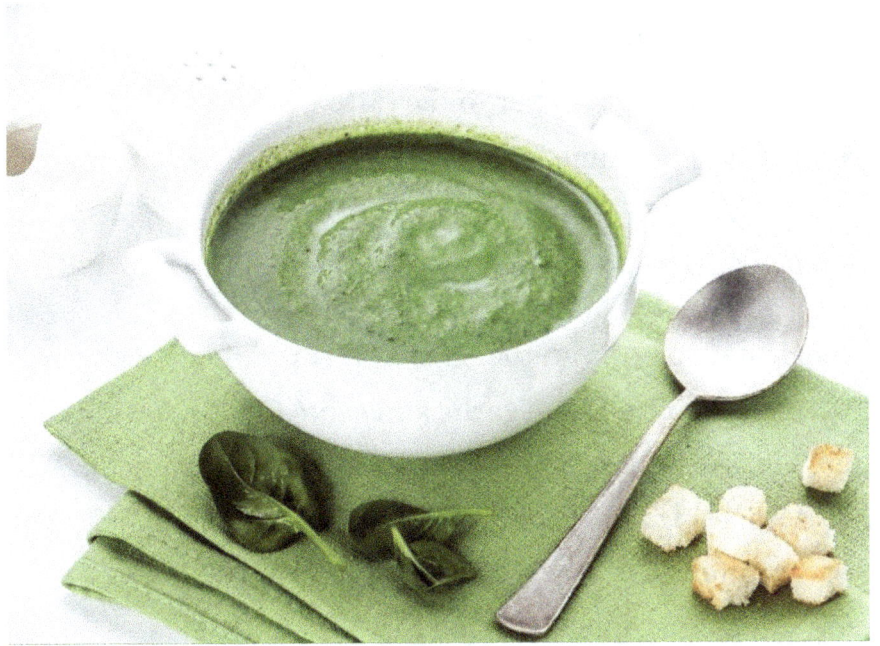

Preparation time: 10 minutes

Cooking time: 20 minutes

Servings: 4

Ingredients:

- 3 shallots, chopped
- 2 garlic cloves, minced
- 1 tablespoon olive oil

- ½ pound broccoli florets
- ½ pound baby spinach
- 4 cups veggie stock
- 1 teaspoon turmeric powder
- Salt and black pepper to the taste
- 1 tablespoon lime juice

Directions:

1. Heat up a pot with the oil over medium-high heat, add the shallots and the garlic and sauté for 5 minutes.
2. Add the broccoli, spinach and the other ingredients, toss, bring to a simmer and cook over medium heat for 15 minutes.
3. Ladle into soup bowls and serve.

Nutrition:

calories 150, fat 3, fiber 1, carbs 3, protein 7

Mushrooms and Chard Soup

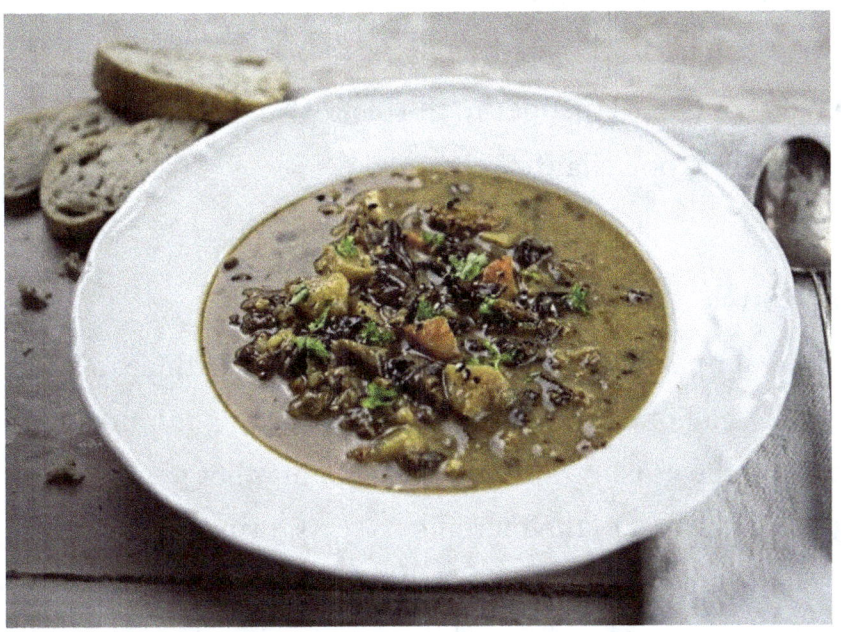

Preparation time: 10 minutes

Cooking time: 30 minutes

Servings: 4

Ingredients:

- 3 cups Swiss chard, chopped
- 6 cups vegetable stock
- 1 cup mushrooms, sliced
- 2 garlic cloves, minced

- 2 scallions, chopped
- 2 tablespoons balsamic vinegar
- 1 tablespoon olive oil
- ¼ cup basil, chopped
- Salt and black pepper to the taste
- 1 tablespoon cilantro, chopped

Directions:

1. Heat up a pot with the oil over medium-high heat, add the scallions and the garlic and sauté for 5 minutes.
2. Add the mushrooms and sauté for another 5 minutes.
3. Add the rest of the ingredients, toss, bring to a simmer and cook over medium heat for 20 minutes more.
4. Ladle the soup into bowls and serve.

Nutrition:

calories 140, fat 4, fiber 2, carbs 4, protein 8

Hot Roasted Peppers Cream

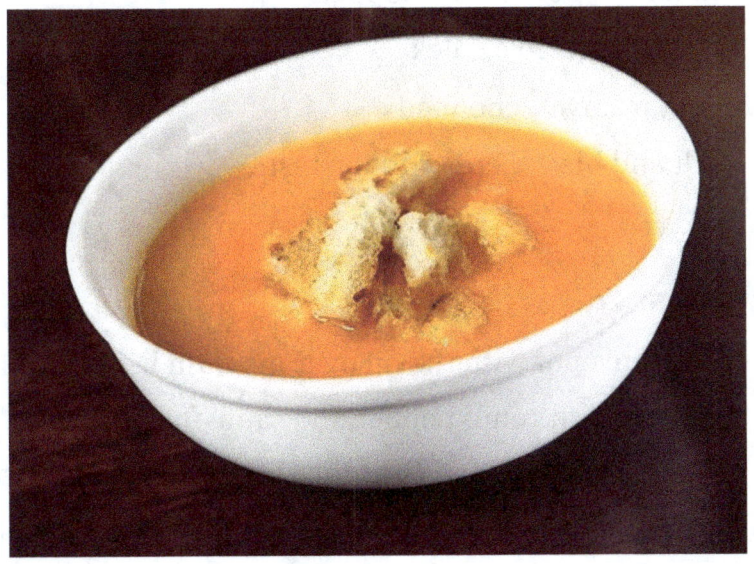

Preparation time: 10 minutes

Cooking time: 30 minutes

Servings: 4

Ingredients:
- 1 red chili pepper, minced
- 4 garlic cloves, minced
- 2 pounds mixed bell peppers, roasted, peeled and chopped
- 4 scallions, chopped

- 1 cup coconut cream
- 2 tablespoons olive oil
- ½ tablespoon basil, chopped
- 4 cups vegetable stock
- ¼ cup chives, chopped
- Salt and black pepper to the taste

Directions:

1. Heat up a pot with the oil over medium heat, add the garlic and the chili pepper and sauté for 5 minutes.
2. Add the peppers and the other ingredients, toss, bring to a simmer and cook over medium heat for 25 minutes.
3. Blend the soup using an immersion blender, divide into bowls and serve.

Nutrition:

calories 140, fat 2, fiber 2, carbs 5, protein 8

Broccoli, Chard and Kale Mix

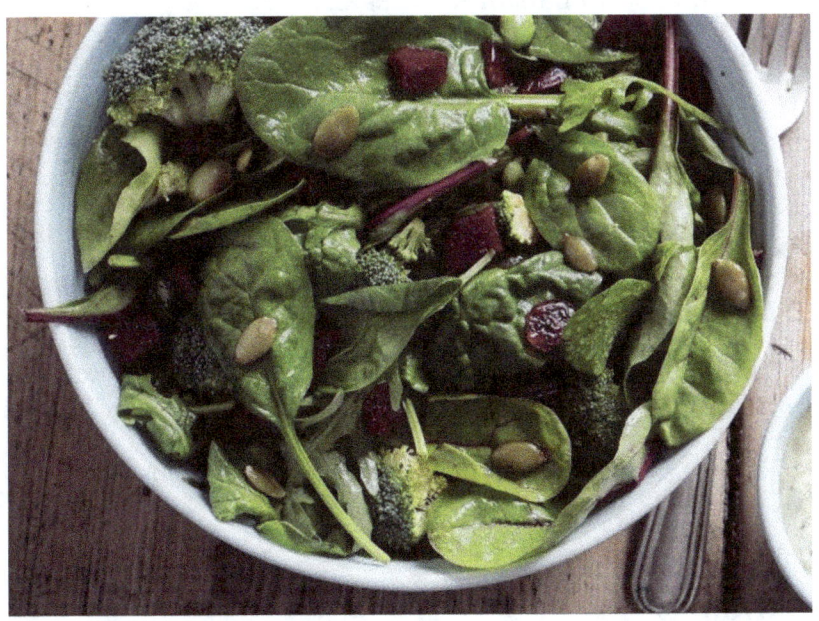

Preparation time: 10 minutes

Cooking time: 20 minutes

Servings: 4

Ingredients:
- 2 cups broccoli florets
- ½ cup kale, torn
- 2 cups red chard, torn
- 4 garlic cloves, minced

- 2 tablespoons olive oil
- 1 tablespoon lemon juice
- 1 tablespoon balsamic vinegar
- ½ cup almonds, sliced
- 1 tablespoon chives, chopped

Directions:

1. In a roasting pan, combine the kale with the chard, broccoli and the other ingredients, toss and bake at 400 degrees F for 20 minutes.
2. Divide everything between plates and serve right away.

Nutrition:

calories 90, fat 1, fiber 3, carbs 7, protein 2

Mashed Cauliflower

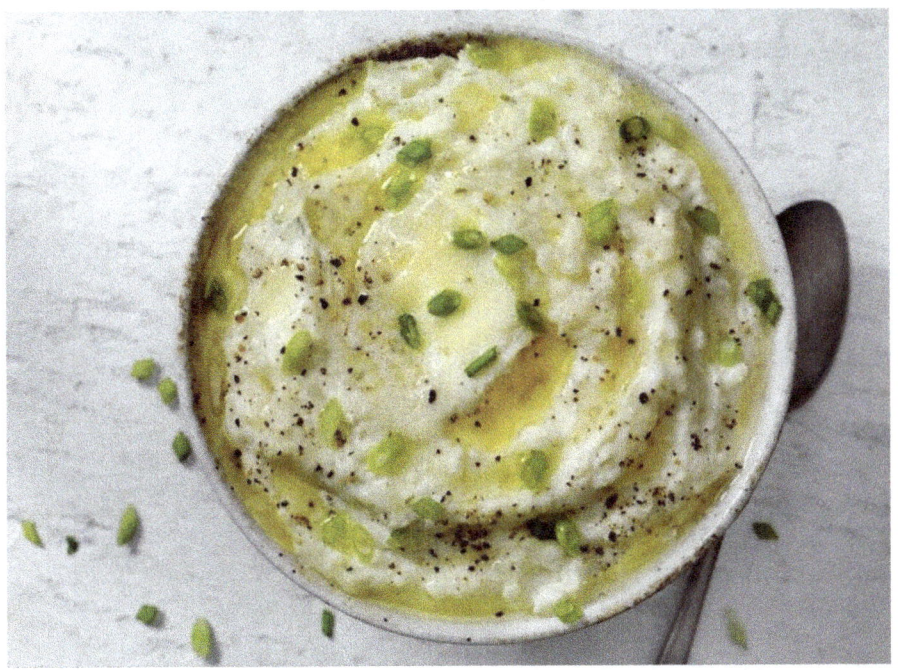

Preparation Time: 10 minutes

Cooking Time: 15 minutes

Servings: 6

Ingredients:

- 2 tablespoons milk
- 2 cauliflower heads, cut into florets
- 4 tablespoons butter

- ½ teaspoon garlic powder
- ½ teaspoon onion powder
- ½ teaspoon sea salt
- ½ teaspoon pepper

Directions:

1. Add your cauliflower to a saucepan filled with enough water to cover the cauliflower.
2. Cook cauliflower over medium heat for 15 minutes. Drain your cauliflower florets and place it in a mixing bowl.
3. Add remaining ingredients to the bowl. Using a blender blend until smooth.
4. Serve and enjoy!

Nutritional Values (Per Serving):

Calories: 120 Fat: 8 g Cholesterol: 21 mg Sugar: 5 g Carbohydrates: 10.9 g Protein: 4.1 g

Simple Grilled Mushrooms

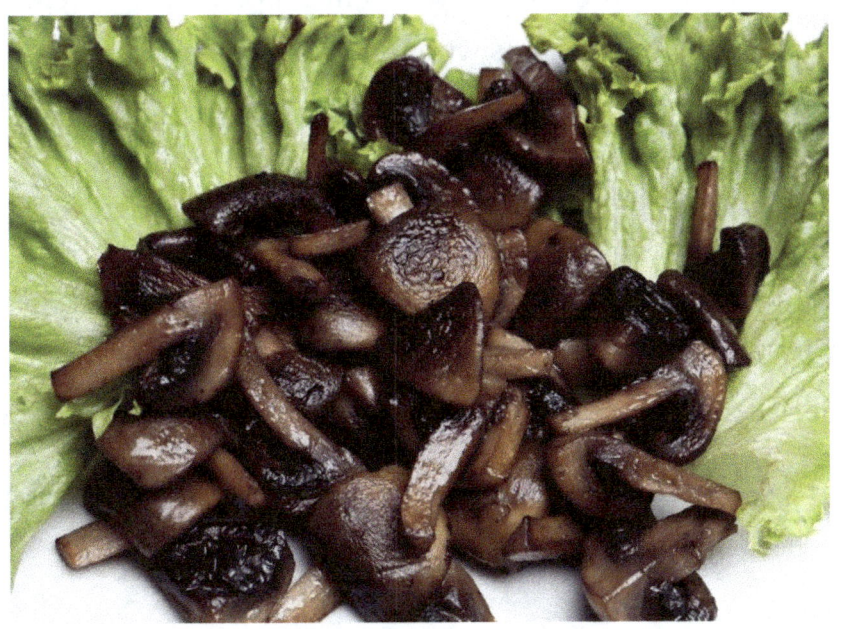

Preparation Time: 25 minutes

Servings: 4

Ingredients:

- 40 cremini mushrooms
- 1/2 tsp black pepper
- 1 tsp sea salt
- 8 tbsp olive oil

Directions:

1. Preheat the oven to 450 °F.
2. Add mushroom and olive oil in a bowl and toss well.
3. Season mushrooms with pepper and salt.
4. Place mushrooms on the rack and grilled in preheated oven for 15 minutes.
5. Serve and enjoy.

Nutritional Value (Amount per Serving):

Calories 295 Fat 28 g Carbohydrates 8 g Sugar 3 g Protein 5 g Cholesterol 0 mg

Braised Seitan with Kelp Noodles

Preparation Time: 10 minutes

Cooking Time: 2 hours 2 minutes

Serving: 4

Ingredients:

- 1 tbsp olive oil
- 2 pieces star anise
- 1 cinnamon stick
- 1-inch ginger, grated
- 2 (23.9oz) kelp noodles, thoroughly rinsed
- 1 ½ lb seitan, cut into strips
- 1 garlic clove, minced
- 3 tbsp tamarind sauce
- 2 tbsp swerve sugar
- ¼ cup red wine
- ¼ cup water
- 4 cups vegetable broth
- For topping:
- 1 cup steamed napa cabbage
- Scallions, thinly sliced

Directions:

1. Heat the olive oil in a medium pot over medium heat and stir-fry the star anise, cinnamon, garlic, and ginger until fragrant, 5 minutes.
2. Mix in the seitan, season with salt, black pepper, and sear on both sides, 10 minutes.
3. In a small bowl, combine the tamarind sauce, swerve sugar, red wine, and water. Pour the mixture into the pot, close the lid, and bring to a boil. Reduce the heat and simmer for 30 to 45 minutes or until the seitan is tender.
4. Strain the pot's content through a colander into a bowl and pour the braising liquid back into the pot. Discard the cinnamon, star anise and set the seitan aside.
5. Add the vegetable broth to the pot and simmer until hot, 10 minutes.
6. Put the kelp noodles into the broth and cook until softened and separated, 5 to 7 minutes.
7. Spoon the noodles with some broth into serving bowls, top with the seitan strips, and then the cabbage and scallions.

Nutrition:

Calories: 311, Total Fat: 18g, Saturated Fat: 6.3g, Total Carbs: 3 g, Dietary Fiber:0 g, Sugar:2 g, Protein:34 g, Sodium:136 mg

Chili Artichokes

Preparation time: 10 minutes

Cooking time: 25 minutes

Servings: 4

Ingredients:

- 2 artichokes, trimmed and halved
- 1 teaspoon chili powder
- 2 tablespoons olive oil
- 2 green chilies, mined
- 1 teaspoon garlic powder
- 1 teaspoon sweet paprika
- A pinch of salt and black pepper
- Juice of 1 lime

Directions:

1. In a roasting pan, combine the artichokes with the chili powder, the chilies and the other ingredients, toss and bake at 380 degrees F for 25 minutes.
2. Divide the artichokes between plates and serve.

Nutrition:

calories 132, fat 2, fiber 2, carbs 4, protein 6

Brussels Sprouts Mix

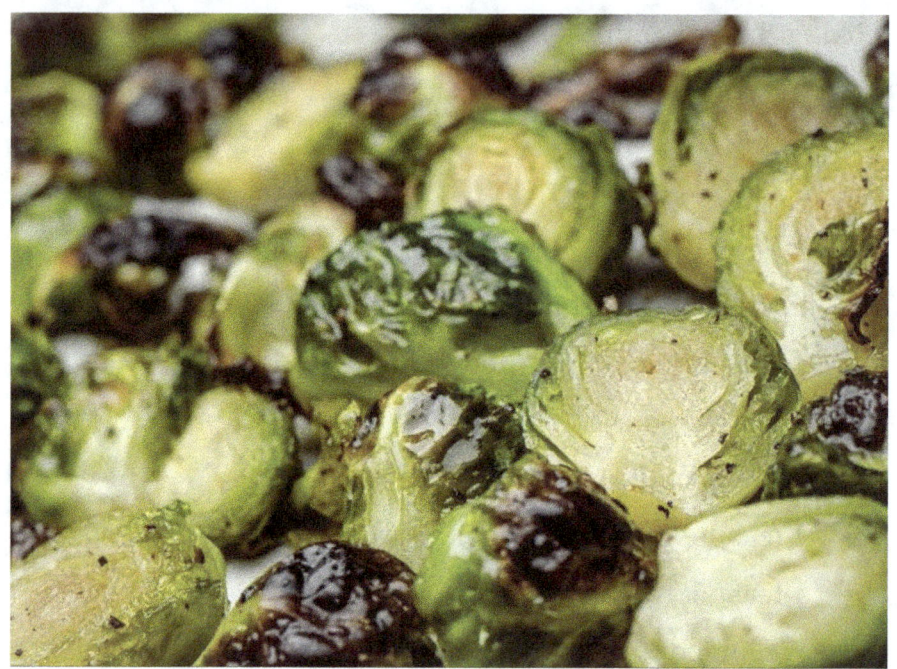

Preparation time: 10 minutes

Cooking time: 20 minutes

Servings: 4

Ingredients:
- 2 tablespoons olive oil
- 1 pound Brussels sprouts, trimmed and halved
- 1 tablespoon ginger, grated

- 1 tablespoon pine nuts
- 1 tablespoon olive oil
- 2 garlic cloves, minced

Directions:

1. Heat up a pan with the oil over medium heat, add the garlic and the ginger and sauté for 2 minutes.
2. Add the Brussels sprouts and the other ingredients, toss, cook for 18 minutes more, divide between plates and serve.

Nutrition:

calories 160, fat 2, fiber 2, carbs 4, protein 5

Tomato Quinoa

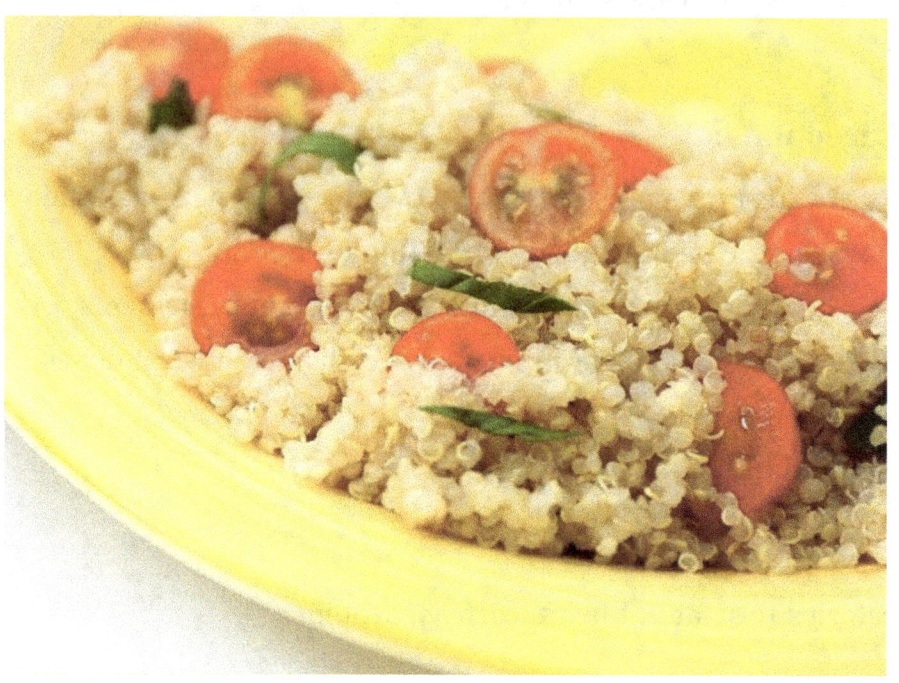

Preparation time: 10 minutes

Cooking time: 25 minutes

Servings: 4

Ingredients:

- 1 cup tomatoes, cubed
- 1 cup quinoa
- 3 cups chicken stock

- 1 tablespoon parsley, chopped
- 1 tablespoon basil, chopped
- 1 teaspoon turmeric powder
- A pinch of salt and black pepper

Directions:

1. In a pot, mix the quinoa with the stock, the tomatoes and the other ingredients, toss, bring to a simmer and cook over medium heat for 25 minutes.
2. Divide everything between plates and serve.

Nutrition:

calories 202, fat 4, fiber 2, carbs 12, protein 10

Mushrooms and Radishes Mix

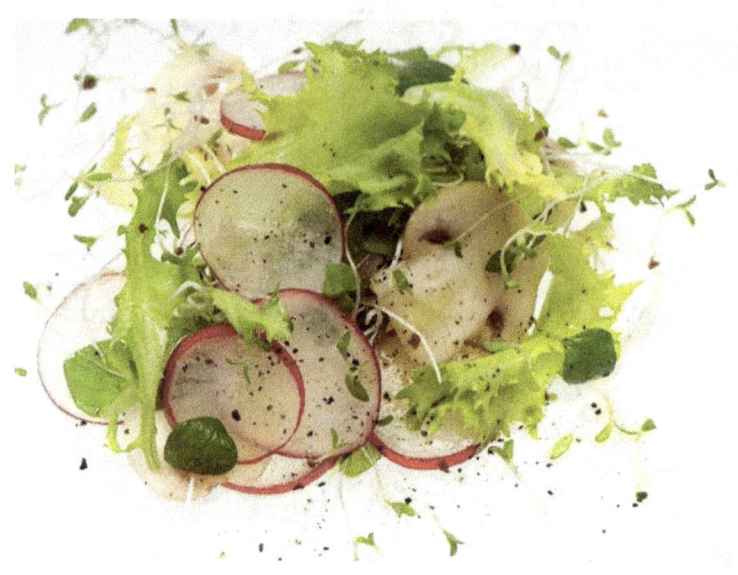

Preparation time: 10 minutes

Cooking time: 25 minutes

Servings: 4

Ingredients:

- 1 pound white mushrooms, halved
- ½ pound radishes, halved
- 4 garlic cloves, minced
- 4 scallions, chopped
- 2 tablespoons olive oil

- ½ cup veggie stock
- 2 tablespoons parsley, chopped
- 1 teaspoon rosemary, dried
- 1 teaspoon coriander, ground
- A pinch of salt and black pepper

Directions:

1. Heat up a pan with the oil over medium heat, add the scallions, garlic, coriander and rosemary, stir and cook for 5 minutes.
2. Add the mushrooms, radishes and the other ingredients, toss, cook over medium heat for 20 minutes, divide between plates and serve as a side dish.

Nutrition:

calories 182, fat 4, fiber 2, carbs 6, protein 8

Simple Sesame Stir-Fry

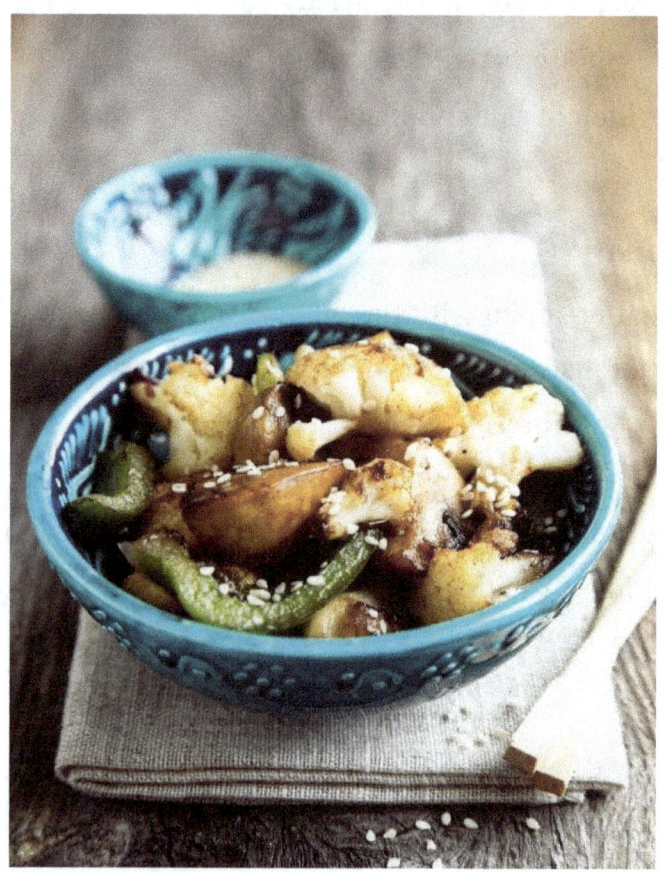

Preparation time: 10 minutes

cooking time: 20 minutes

servings: 4

Ingredients

- 1 cup quinoa
- 2 cups water
- 1 head broccoli
- 1 cup snow peas, or snap peas, ends trimmed and cut in half
- 1 to 2 teaspoons untoasted sesame oil, or olive oil
- 1 cup frozen shelled edamame beans, or peas
- 2 cups chopped Swiss chard, or other large-leafed green
- 2 scallions, chopped
- 2 tablespoons water
- Pinch sea salt
- 1 teaspoon toasted sesame oil
- 1 tablespoon tamari, or soy sauce
- 2 tablespoons sesame seeds

Directions

1. Put the quinoa, water, and sea salt in a medium pot, bring it to a boil for a minute, then turn to low and simmer, covered, for 20 minutes. The quinoa is fully cooked when you see the swirl of the grains with a translucent center, and it is fluffy. Do not stir the quinoa while it is cooking.
2. Meanwhile, cut the broccoli into bite-size florets, cutting and pulling apart from the stem. Also chop the

stem into bite-size pieces. Heat a large skillet to high, and sauté the broccoli in the untoasted sesame oil, with a pinch of salt to help it soften. Keep this moving continuously, so that it doesn't burn, and add an extra drizzle of oil if needed as you add the rest of the vegetables. Add the snow peas next, continuing to stir. Add the edamame until they thaw. Add the Swiss chard and scallions at the same time, tossing for only a minute to wilt. Then add 2 tablespoons of water to the hot skillet so that it sizzles and finishes the vegetables with a quick steam.

3. Dress with the toasted sesame oil and tamari, and toss one last time. Remove from the heat immediately. Serve a scoop of cooked quinoa, topped with stir-fry and sprinkled with some sesame seeds, and an extra drizzle of tamari and/or toasted sesame oil if you like.

Nutrition:

Calories: 334; Total fat: 13g; Carbs: 42g; Fiber: 9g; Protein: 17g

Minted Peas

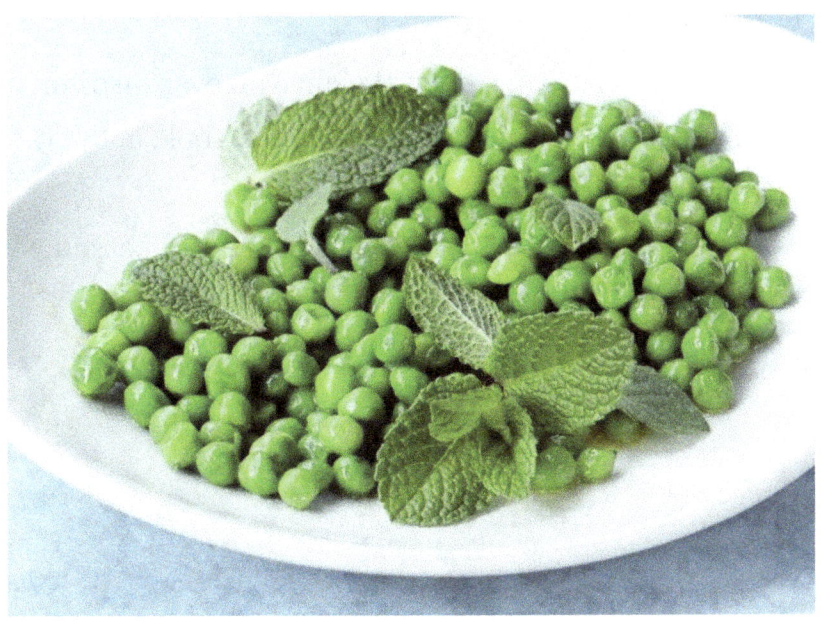

Preparation time: 5 minutes

cooking time: 5 minutes

servings: 4

Ingredients

- 1 tablespoon olive oil
- 4 cups peas, fresh or frozen (not canned
- freshly ground black pepper
- ½ teaspoon sea salt

- 3 tablespoons chopped fresh mint

Directions

1. In a large sauté pan, heat the olive oil over medium-high heat until hot. Add the peas and cook, about 5 minutes.
2. Remove the pan from heat. Stir in the salt, season with pepper, and stir in the mint.
3. Serve hot.

Basic Baked Potatoes

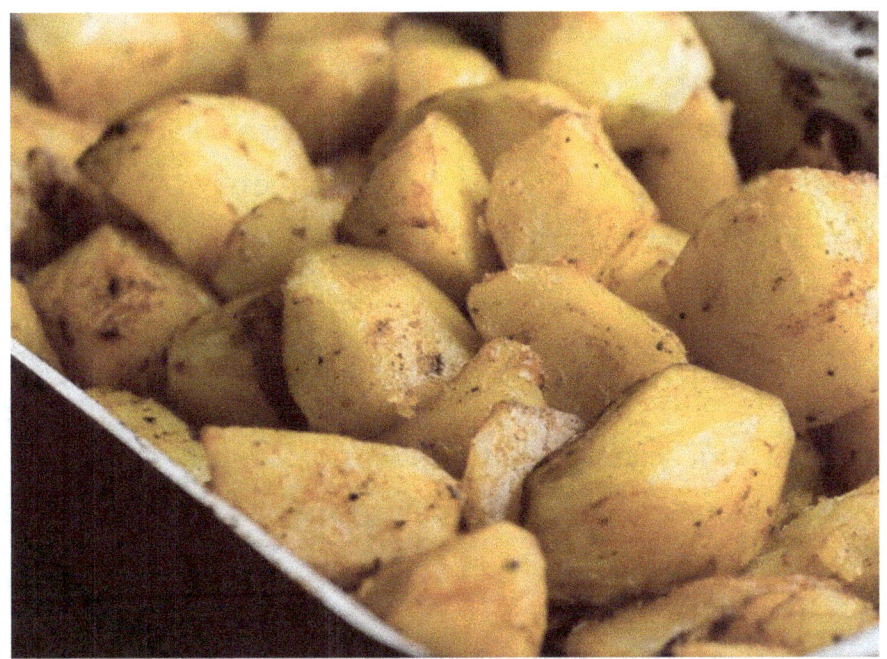

Preparation time: 5 minutes

cooking time: 60 minutes

servings: 5

Ingredients
1. 5 medium Russet potatoes or a variety of potatoes, washed and patted dry
2. 1 to 2 tablespoons extra-virgin olive oil or aquafaba (see tip

3. ¼ teaspoon freshly ground black pepper
4. ¼ teaspoon salt

Directions

1. Preheat the oven to 400°F. Pierce each potato several times with a fork or a knife. Brush the olive oil over the potatoes, then rub each with a pinch of the salt and a pinch of the pepper.
2. Place the potatoes on a baking sheet and bake for 50 to 60 minutes, until tender. Place the potatoes on a baking rack and cool completely. Transfer to an air-tight container or 5 single-serving containers. Let cool before sealing the lids.

Nutrition:

Calories: 171; Fat: 3g; Protein: 4g; Carbohydrates: 34g; Fiber: 5g; Sugar: 3g; Sodium: 129mg

Orange-Dressed Asparagus

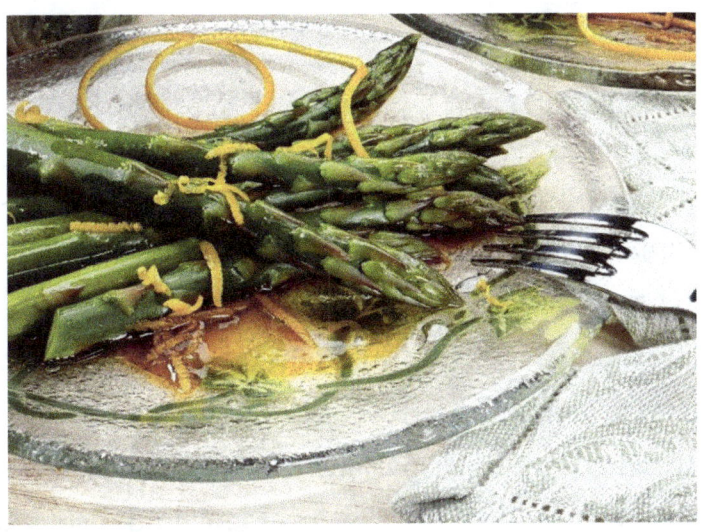

Preparation time: 5 minutes

cooking time: 10 minutes

servings: 4

Ingredients

- 1 medium shallot, minced
- 2 teaspoons orange zest
- 1/3 cup fresh orange juice
- 1 pound asparagus, tough ends trimmed
- 1 tablespoon fresh lemon juice
- 2 tablespoons olive oil

- Pinch sugar
- Salt and freshly ground black pepper

Directions

1. In a small bowl, combine the shallot, orange zest, orange juice, lemon juice, sugar, and oil. Add salt and pepper to taste and mix well. Set aside to allow flavors to blend, for 5 to 10 minutes.
2. Steam the asparagus until just tender, 4 to 5 minutes. If serving hot, arrange on a serving platter and drizzle the dressing over the asparagus. Serve at once.
3. If serving chilled, run the asparagus under cold water to stop the cooking process and retain the color. Drain on paper towels, then cover and refrigerate until chilled, about 1 hour. To serve, arrange the asparagus on a serving platter and drizzle with the dressing.

Broccoli With Almonds

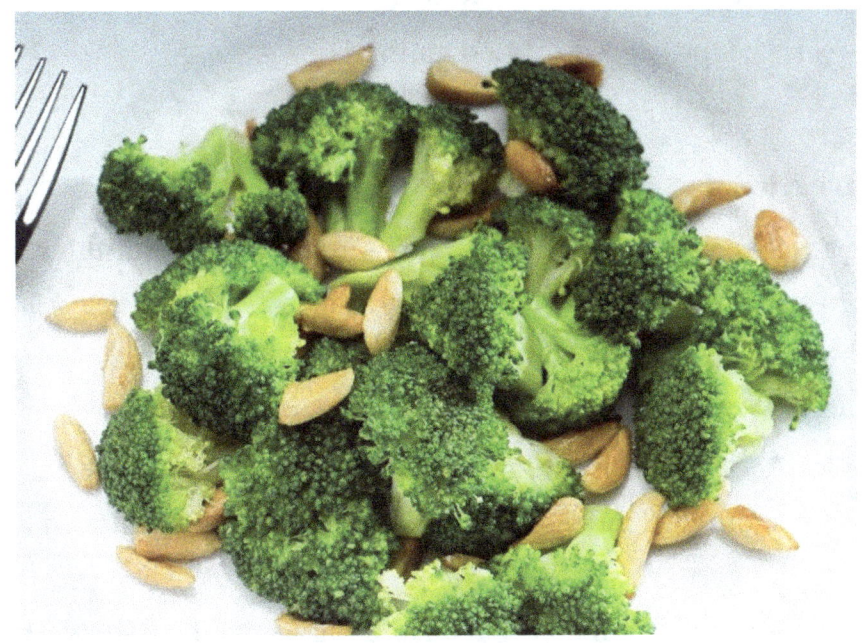

Preparation time: 5 minutes

cooking time: 15 minutes

servings: 4

Ingredients

- 1 pound broccoli, cut into small florets
- 1 cup thinly sliced white mushrooms
- 2 tablespoons olive oil
- 3 garlic cloves, minced

- 1/4 cup dry white wine
- 2 tablespoons minced fresh parsley
- Salt and freshly ground black pepper
- 1/2 cup slivered toasted almonds

Directions

1. Steam the broccoli until just tender, about 5 minutes. Run under cold water and set aside.
2. In a large skillet, heat 1 tablespoon of the oil over medium heat.
3. Add the garlic and mushrooms and cook until soft, about 5 minutes. Add the wine and cook 1 minute longer.
4. Add the steamed broccoli and parsley and season with salt and pepper to taste. Cook until the liquid is evaporated and the broccoli is hot, about 3 minutes.
5. Transfer to a serving bowl, drizzle with the remaining 1 tablespoon oil and the almonds, and toss to coat. Serve immediately.

Roasted Bell Peppers Soup

Preparation time: 10 minutes

Cooking time: 15 minutes

Servings: 6

Ingredients:

- 12 ounces roasted bell peppers, seeded and chopped
- 2 tablespoons olive oil
- 2 garlic cloves, peeled and minced
- 29 ounces canned chicken stock
- 7 ounces water
- ⅔ cup heavy cream
- 1 onion, peeled and chopped
- Salt and ground black pepper, to taste
- ¼ cup Parmesan cheese, grated
- 2 celery stalks, chopped

Directions:

1. Heat up a pot with the oil over medium heat, add the onion, garlic, celery, and some salt, and pepper, stir, and cook for 8 minutes.

2. Add the bell peppers, water, and stock, stir, bring to a boil, cover, reduce the heat, and simmer for 5 minutes.
3. Use an immersion blender to puree the soup, then add more salt, pepper, and cream, stir, bring to a boil, and take off the heat.
4. Ladle into bowls, sprinkle Parmesan cheese, and serve.

Nutrition:

Calories - 176, Fat - 13, Fiber - 1, Carbs - 4, Protein - 6

Cream Of Artichoke Soup

Preparation time: 10 minutes

cooking time: 20 minutes

servings: 4

Ingredients

- 1 tablespoon olive oil
- 2 medium shallots, chopped
- 3 cups vegetable broth, homemade (see Light Vegetable Broth or store-bought, or water
- 2 (10-ouncepackages frozen artichoke hearts, thawed
- 1 teaspoon fresh lemon juice
- 1/3 cup almond butter
- 1/8 teaspoon ground cayenne
- 1 cup plain unsweetened soy milk
- Salt
- 1 tablespoon snipped fresh chives, for garnish
- 2 tablespoons sliced toasted almonds, for garnish

Directions

1. In a large soup pot, heat the oil over medium heat. Add the shallots, cover, and cook until softened.

2. Uncover and stir in the artichoke hearts, broth, lemon juice, and salt to taste.
3. Bring to a boil, then reduce heat to low and simmer, uncovered, until the artichokes are tender, about 20 minutes.
4. Add the almond butter and cayenne to the artichoke mixture. Puree in a high-speed blender or food processor, in batches if necessary, and return to the pot.
5. Stir in the soy milk and taste, adjusting seasonings if necessary. Simmer the soup over medium heat until hot, about 5 minutes.
6. Ladle into bowls, sprinkle with chives and almonds, and serve.

Butternut Soup With A Swirl Of Cranberry

Preparation time: 10 minutes

cooking time: 30 minutes

servings: 4 to 6

Ingredients

- 2 tablespoons olive oil
- 1 medium russet potato, peeled and chopped
- 1 medium onion, chopped
- 1 medium carrot, chopped
- 1/2 teaspoon ground allspice
- 1/4 teaspoon ground ginger
- 4 cups vegetable broth, homemade (see Light Vegetable Broth or store-bought, or water
- 3 pounds butternut squash, peeled, seeded, and cut into 1-inch pieces
- Salt
- 1/2 cup whole berry cranberry sauce, homemade or canned
- 2 tablespoons fresh orange juice

Directions

1. In a large soup pot, heat the oil over medium heat. Add the onion and carrot, cover, and cook, stirring occasionally, until softened, about 5 minutes. Stir in the allspice, ginger, potato, squash, broth, and salt to taste. Simmer, uncovered, until the vegetables are very soft, about 30 minutes.
2. While the soup is cooking, puree the cranberry sauce and orange juice in a blender or food processor. Run the pureed cranberry sauce through a strainer and discard solids. Set aside.
3. When the soup is done cooking, puree it in the pot with an immersion blender or in a blender or food processor, in batches if necessary, and return to the pot. Reheat the soup and taste, adjusting seasonings if necessary.
4. Ladle into bowls, swirl a tablespoon or so of the reserved cranberry puree into the center of each bowl, and serve.

Mom's Creamy Broccoli and Rice Bake

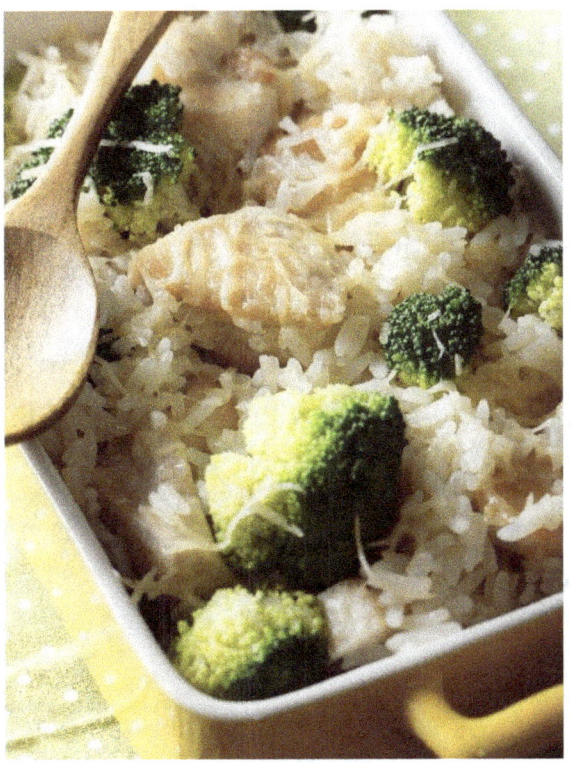

Preparation Time: 10 Minutes

Cooking Time: 40 Minutes

Servings: 7

Ingredients

- 2 cups cooked brown rice
- ½ cup chopped onion

- 1 (12-ounce) bag frozen broccoli florets, chopped, or 2 cups chopped fresh broccoli florets
- 1 celery stalk, thinly sliced
- 1 batch Easy Vegan Cheese Sauce

Directions

- Preparing the Ingredients.
- Preheat the oven to 425 °F.
- In a large bowl, mix together the rice, broccoli, onion, celery, and cheese sauce. Transfer to a 2-quart or 8-inch-square baking dish.
- Bake for 40 minutes, or until the top has started to brown slightly.

Mexican Fideo Soup With Pinto Beans

Preparation Time: 5 Minutes

Cooking Time: 25 Minutes

Servings: 4

Ingredients

- 3 tablespoons olive oil
- 1 medium onion, chopped
- 3 garlic cloves, chopped
- 1 (14.5-ounce) can crushed tomatoes
- 8 ounces fideo, vermicelli, or angel hair pasta, broken into 2-inch pieces
- 1½ cups cooked or 1 (15.5-ounce) can pinto beans, rinsed and drained
- 1 (4-ounce) can chopped hot or mild green chiles
- 1 teaspoon ground cumin
- ½ teaspoon dried oregano
- 6 cups vegetable broth, homemade (see Light Vegetable Broth) or store-bought, or water
- Salt and freshly ground black pepper
- ¼ cup chopped fresh cilantro, for garnish

Directions

1. In a large soup pot, heat 1 tablespoon of the oil over medium heat. Add the onion, cover, and cook until soft, about 10 minutes. Stir in the garlic and cook 1 minute longer. Remove the onion mixture with a slotted spoon and set aside.
2. In the same pot, heat the remaining 2 tablespoons of oil over medium heat, add the noodles, and cook until golden, stirring frequently 5 to 7 minutes. Be careful not to burn the noodles.
3. Stir in the tomatoes, beans, chiles, cumin, oregano, broth, and salt and pepper to taste. Stir in the onion mixture and simmer until the vegetables and noodles are tender, 10 to 15 minutes. Ladle into soup bowls, garnish with cilantro, and serve.

Senegalese Soup

Preparation Time: 5 Minutes

Cooking Time: 40 Minutes

Servings: 4

Ingredients

- 1 tablespoon canola or grapeseed oil
- 1 medium onion, chopped
- 1 medium carrot, chopped
- 2 teaspoons tomato paste
- 1 cup plain unsweetened soy milk
- 1 garlic clove, minced
- 3 Granny Smith apples, peeled, cored, and chopped
- 2 tablespoons hot or mild curry powder
- 3 cups light vegetable broth, homemade (see Light Vegetable Broth) or store-bought, or water
- Salt
- 4 teaspoons mango chutney, homemade or store-bought, for garnish

Directions

1. In a large soup pot, heat the oil over medium heat. Add the onion, carrot, and garlic. Cover and cook until

softened, about 10 minutes. Add the apples and continue to cook, uncovered, occasionally stirring, until the apples begin to soften, about 5 minutes. Add the curry powder and cook, stirring, 1 minute. Stir in the tomato paste, broth, and salt to taste. Simmer, uncovered, for 30 minutes.

2. Puree the soup in the pot with an immersion blender or in a blender or food processor, in batches if necessary. Pour the soup into a large container, stir in the soy milk, cover, and refrigerate until chilled, about 3 hours.
3. Ladle the soup into bowls, garnish each with a teaspoonful of chutney, and serve.

Greek Potato Salad

Preparation Time: 10 Minutes

Cooking Time: 20 Minutes

Servings: 4

Ingredients

- 6 potatoes, scrubbed or peeled and chopped
- ¼ cup olive oil
- 2 tablespoons apple cider vinegar
- 2 tablespoons freshly squeezed lemon juice
- ½ cucumber, chopped
- 1 teaspoon dried herbs
- ¼ red onion, diced
- Salt
- ¼ cup chopped pitted black olives
- Freshly ground black pepper

Directions

1. Put the potatoes in a large pot, add a pinch of salt, and pour in enough water to cover. Bring the water to a boil over high heat. Cook the potatoes for 15 to 20 minutes, until soft. Drain and set aside to cool. (Alternatively, put the potatoes in a large microwave-safe dish with a

bit of water. Cover and heat on high power for 10 minutes.)
2. In a large bowl, whisk together the olive oil, vinegar, lemon juice, and dried herbs. Toss the cucumber, red onion, and olives with the dressing. Add the cooked, cooled potatoes, and toss to combine. Taste and season with salt and pepper as needed. Store leftovers in an air-tight container in the refrigerator for up to 1 week.

Nutrition, per Serving

Calories: 358; Protein: 5g; Total fat: 16g; Saturated fat: 2g; Carbohydrates: 52g; Fiber: 5g

Quinoa Salad With Black Beans And Tomatoes

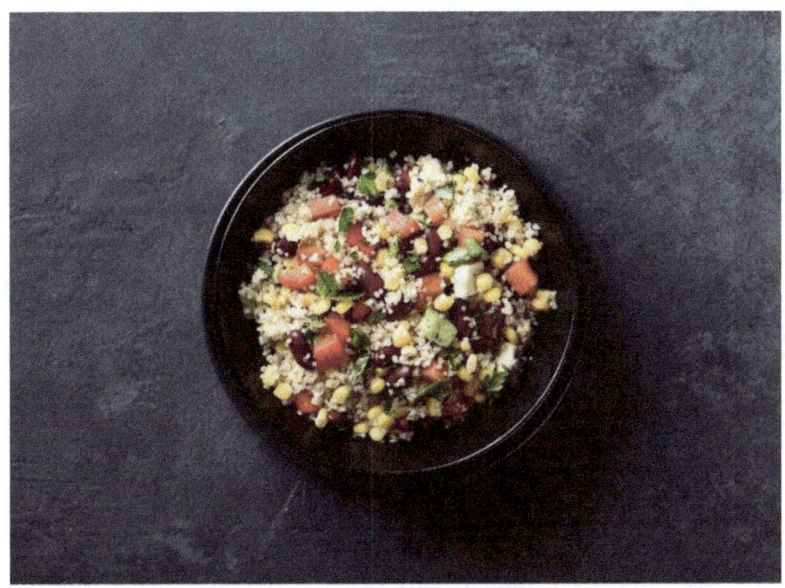

Preparation Time: 5 Minutes

Cooking Time: 20 Minutes

Servings:4

Ingredients

- 3 cups water
- 1 1/2 cups quinoa, well rinsed
- Salt

- 1/4 cup olive oil
- 1 1/2 cups cooked or 1 (15.5-ounce) can black beans, drained and rinsed
- 4 ripe plum tomatoes, cut into 1/4-inch dice
- 1/3 cup minced red onion
- 1/4 cup chopped fresh parsley
- 2 tablespoons sherry vinegar
- 1/4 teaspoon freshly ground black pepper

Directions

1. In a large saucepan, bring the water to boil over high heat. Add the quinoa, salt the water, and return to a boil. Reduce heat to low, cover, and simmer until the water is absorbed, about 20 minutes.
2. Transfer the cooked quinoa to a large bowl. Add the black beans, tomatoes, onion, and parsley.
3. In a small bowl, combine the olive oil, vinegar, salt to taste, and pepper. Pour the dressing over the salad and toss well to combine. Cover and set aside for 20 minutes before serving.

Balsamic Pearl Onions Bowls

Preparation time: 5 minutes

Cooking time: 15 minutes

Servings: 4

Ingredients:

- 1 pound pearl onions, peeled
- 2 tablespoons avocado oil
- 4 tablespoons balsamic vinegar
- A pinch of salt and black pepper
- 1 tablespoon chives, chopped

Directions:

1. Heat up a pan with the oil over medium heat, add the pearl onions, salt, pepper and the other ingredients, cook for 15 minutes, divide into bowls and serve as a snack.

Nutrition:

calories 120, fat 2, fiber 1, carbs 2, protein 2

Hot Eggplant and Broccoli Spread

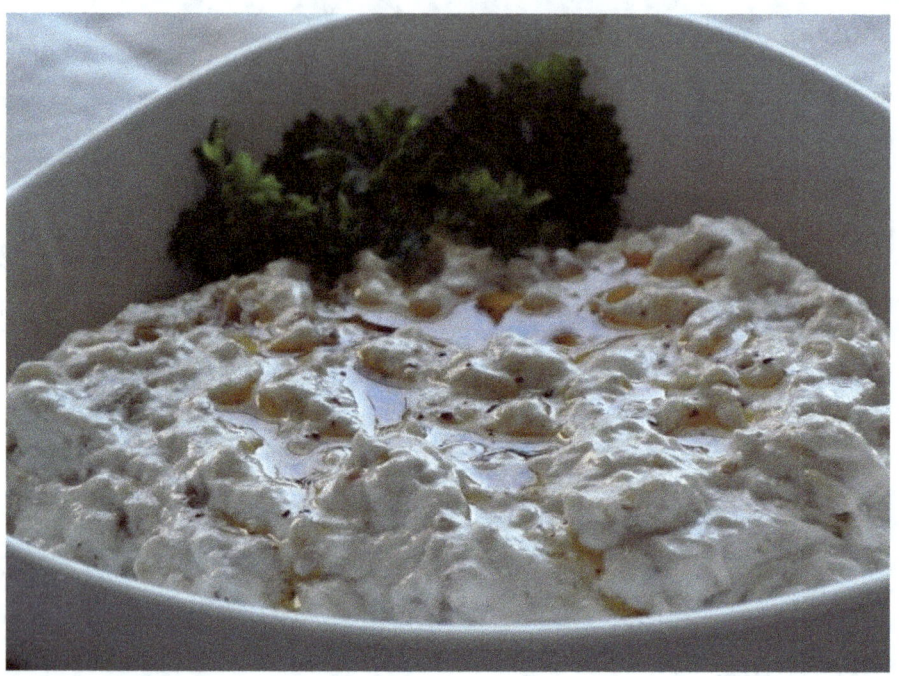

Preparation time: 10 minutes

Cooking time: 25 minutes

Servings: 8

Ingredients:

- ½ cup walnuts, chopped
- 1 cup broccoli florets
- 2 eggplants, cubed

- 1 cup coconut cream
- 1 teaspoon hot paprika
- ½ teaspoon garlic powder
- 1 teaspoon cumin, ground
- ½ teaspoon chili powder
- A pinch of salt and black pepper
- ½ teaspoon rosemary, dried

Directions:
1. Heat up a pan with the cream over medium heat, add the walnuts, eggplants, broccoli and the other ingredients, stir, cook for 25 minutes and transfer to a blender.
2. Pulse well, divide into bowls and serve as a party spread.

Nutrition:
calories 192, fat 5, fiber 7, carbs 9, protein 8

Coconut Cashew Dip

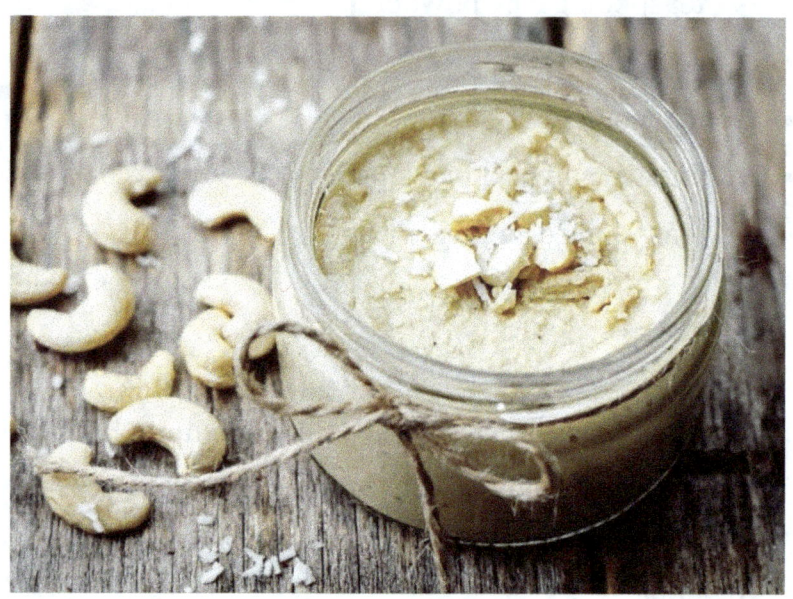

Preparation time: 10 minutes

Cooking time: 30 minutes

Servings: 4

Ingredients:

- 2 tablespoons cashew cheese, shredded
- ½ cup coconut cream
- 1 cup cashews, chopped
- 1 teaspoon balsamic vinegar
- 1 tablespoon chives, chopped

- A pinch of salt and black pepper

Directions:

1. In a pot, combine the cream with the cashew, cashew cheese and the other ingredients, stir, cook over medium heat for 30 minutes and transfer to a blender.
2. Pulse well, divide into bowls and serve.

Nutrition:

calories 100, fat 2, fiber 1, carbs 6, protein 6

Pomegranate Dip

Preparation time: 10 minutes

Cooking time: 0 minutes

Servings: 6

Ingredients:

- 2 cups coconut cream
- 2 tablespoons walnuts, chopped
- ½ cup pomegranate seeds
- 2 tablespoons mint, chopped
- A pinch of salt and white pepper
- 2 tablespoons olive oil

Directions:

1. In a blender, combine the cream with the pomegranate seeds and the other ingredients, pulse well, divide into bowls and serve cold.

Nutrition:

calories 294, fat 18, fiber 1, carbs 21, protein 10

Creamy Blackberry Cinnamon Smoothie

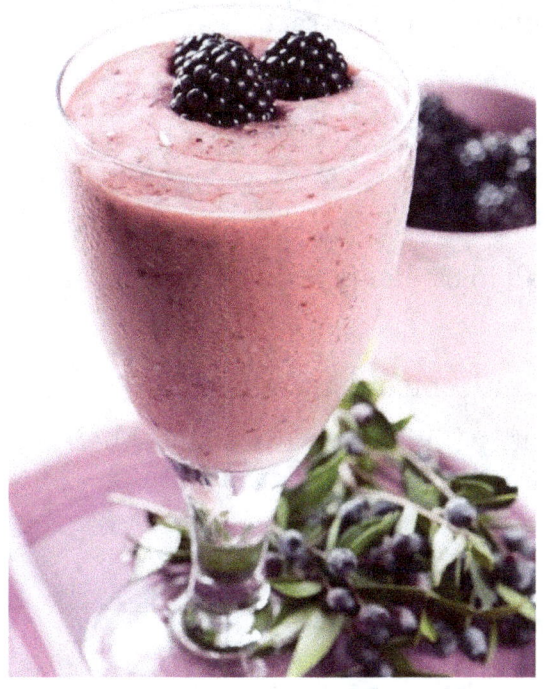

Preparation Time: 3 minutes

Cooking Time: 0 minutes

Servings: 3

Ingredients

- 1 c. frozen blackberries
- 1 c. unsweetened vanilla almond milk

- 2 tsp. ground cinnamon
- 1 tbsp. arrowroot powder
- ½ c. full fat vanilla yogurt
- 1 tsp. pure vanilla extract
- ½ c. water

Directions:

1. Place all ingredients from the list in your high-speed blender.
2. Blend until smooth and creamy.
3. Decorate with fresh or frozen blackberries and serve.
4. Enjoy!

Nutrition:

Calories: 83.78, Fat: 1.42g, Carbs: 8.56g, Protein: 2.97g

Beans and Spinach Tacos

Preparation Time: 10 minutes

Cooking Time: 15 minutes

Servings: 4

Ingredients:

- 12 ounces spinach
- 4 tablespoons cooked kidney beans
- 1 medium tomato, chopped
- ½ of medium red onion, peeled, chopped
- ½ teaspoon minced garlic
- 3 tablespoons chopped parsley
- ½ of avocado, sliced
- 2 tablespoons olive oil
- 4 slices of vegan brie cheese
- 4 tortillas, about 6-inches
- ½ teaspoon ground black pepper
- 1 teaspoon salt

Directions:

1. Take a skillet pan, place it over medium heat, add oil and when hot, add onion and cook for 10 minutes until softened.

2. Then stir in spinach, cook for 4 minutes until its leaf's wilts, then drain it and distribute evenly between tortillas.
3. Top evenly with remaining ingredients, season with black pepper and salt, drizzle with lemon juice and then serve.

Nutrition:

Calories: 8 Cal, Fat: 6 g, Carbs: 34 g, Protein: 9.9 g, Fiber: 10 g

Crispy Kale Chips

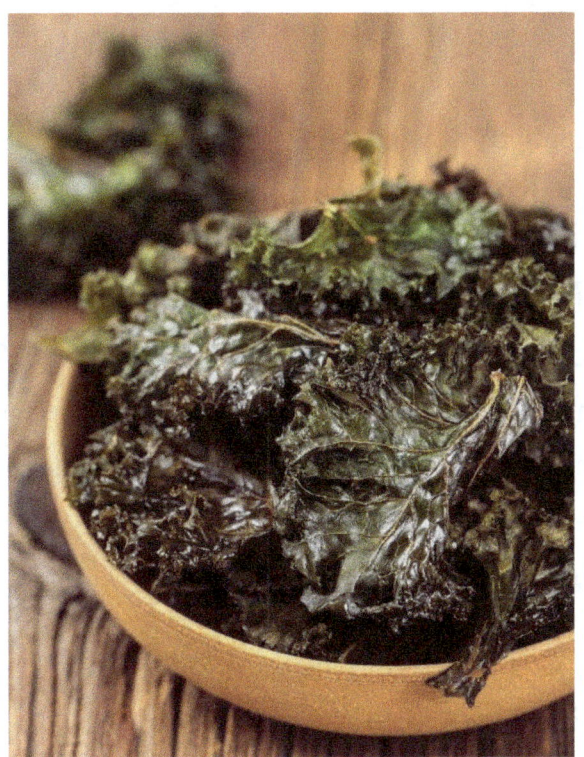

Preparation Time: 10 minutes

Cooking Time: 12 minutes

Servings: 2

Ingredients:
- 1 cup kale, fresh

- 2 teaspoons garlic seasoning
- 2 teaspoons sesame seeds, toasted

Directions:

1. Preheat your oven to 325° Fahrenheit. Spray baking dish with cooking spray and set aside.
2. Wash kale and pat dry with paper towel.
3. Cut the kale and tear into pieces and place in a baking dish.
4. Spray kale with cooking spray.
5. Sprinkle sesame seeds and seasoning over the kale.
6. Bake in preheated oven for 12 minutes.
7. Serve and enjoy.

Nutrition:

Calories: 55 Carbohydrates: 5.2 g Fat: 2.3 g Sugar: 0 g Cholesterol: 0 mg Protein: 2 g

Chinese Soup And Ginger Sauce

Preparation time: 10 minutes

Cooking time: 8 hours

Servings: 6

Ingredients:

- 2 celery stalks, chopped
- 1 yellow onion, chopped
- 1 cup carrot, chopped
- 8 ounces water chestnuts
- 8 ounces canned bamboo shoots, drained
- 2 teaspoons garlic, minced
- 2 teaspoons ginger paste
- ½ teaspoon red pepper flakes
- 3 tablespoons coconut aminos
- 1-quart veggie stock
- 2 bunches bok choy, chopped
- 5 ounces white mushrooms, sliced
- 8 ounces tofu, drained and cubed
- 1 ounce snow peas, cut into small pieces
- 6 scallions, chopped
- For the ginger sauce:
- 1 teaspoon sesame oil

- 2 tablespoons ginger paste
- 2 tablespoons agave syrup
- 2 tablespoon coconut aminos

Directions:

1. In your slow cooker, mix onion with carrot, celery, chestnuts, bamboo shoots, garlic paste, 2 teaspoons ginger paste, pepper flakes, 3 tablespoons coconut aminos, stock, bok choy, mushrooms, tofu, snow peas and scallions, stir, cover and cook on Low for 8 hours.
2. In a bowl, mix 2 tablespoons ginger paste with agave syrup, 2 tablespoons coconut aminos and sesame oil and whisk well.
3. Ladle Chinese soup into bowls, add ginger sauce on top and serve.
4. Enjoy!

Nutrition:

calories 300, fat 4, fiber 6, carbs 19, protein 4

Eggplant Salad

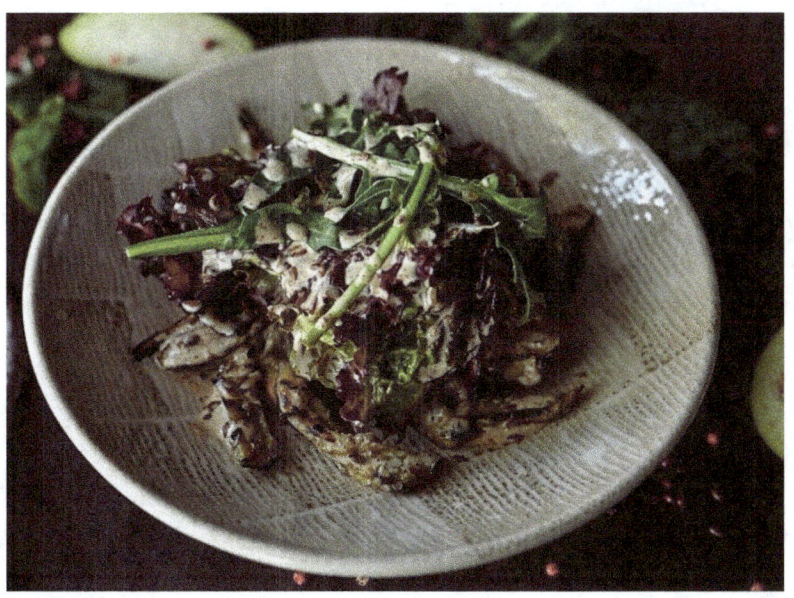

Preparation time: 10 minutes

Cooking time: 8 hours

Servings: 4

Ingredients:

- 24 ounces canned tomatoes, chopped
- 2 red bell peppers, chopped
- 1 big eggplant, roughly chopped
- 1 red onion, chopped

- 1 tablespoons parsley, chopped
- 1 tablespoon smoked paprika
- 2 teaspoons cumin, ground
- Salt and black pepper to the taste
- Juice of 1 lemon

Directions:

1. In your slow cooker, mix tomatoes with onion, bell peppers, eggplant, smoked paprika, cumin, salt, pepper and lemon juice, stir, cover and cook on Low for 8 hours
2. Add parsley, stir, divide into bowls and serve cold as a dinner salad.
3. Enjoy!

Nutrition:

calories 251, fat 4, fiber 6, carbs 8, protein 3

Zucchini & Ricotta Tart

Preparation Time: 25 minutes

Cooking Time: about 1 hour

Servings: 8

Ingredients:

For the crust:

- 1¾ cups almond flour
- ¼ cup melted butter
- 1 tablespoon coconut flour
- ½ teaspoon garlic powder
- ¼ teaspoon salt

For the filling:

- 3 large eggs
- 1 medium-large zucchini, thinly sliced cross-wise (use a mandolin if you have one)
- ½ teaspoon salt
- 8 ounces ricotta
- ¼ cup whipping cream
- 2 cloves garlic, minced
- 1 teaspoon fresh dill, minced
- Additional salt and pepper to taste

- ½ cup shredded parmesan

Directions:

To make the crust:

1. Preheat oven to 325 °F.
2. Lightly spray 9-inch ceramic or glass tart pan with cooking spray.
3. Combine the almond flour, coconut flour, garlic powder and salt in a large bowl.
4. Add the butter and stir until dough resembles coarse crumbs.
5. Press the dough gently into the tart pan, trimming away any excess.
6. Bake 15 minutes then remove from the oven and let cool.

To make the filling:

7. While crust is baking, put the zucchini slices into a colander and sprinkle each layer with a little salt. Let sit and drain for 30 minutes.
8. Place salted zucchini between double layers of paper towels and gently press down to remove any excess water.

9. Place the ricotta, eggs, whipping cream, garlic, dill, salt and pepper in a bowl and stir well to combine. Add almost all the zucchini slices, reserving about 25-30 for layering on top.
10. Transfer mixture into cooled crust. Top with the remaining zucchini slices, slightly overlapping.
11. Sprinkle with parmesan cheese.
12. Bake 60 to 70 minutes or until center is no longer wobbly and a toothpick comes out clean.
13. Cut into slices and serve.

Nutrition:

Calories: 302, Total Fats: 25.2g, Carbohydrates: 7.9g, Fiber: 3.1g, Protein: 12.4g

Pumpkin Pie Cups (Pressure cooker)

Preparation time: 5 minutes

Servings: 4-6

Ingredients

- 1 cup canned pumpkin purée
- 1 cup nondairy milk
- 6 tablespoons unrefined sugar or pure maple syrup (less if using sweetened milk), plus more for sprinkling
- ½ teaspoon pumpkin pie spice
- ¼ cup spelt flour or all-purpose flour
- Pinch salt

Directions

1. In a medium bowl, stir together the pumpkin, milk, sugar, flour, pumpkin pie spice, and salt. Pour the mixture into 4 heat-proof ramekins. Sprinkle a bit more sugar on the top of each, if you like. Put a trivet in the bottom of your electric pressure cooker's cooking pot and pour in a cup or two of water. Place the ramekins onto the trivet, stacking them if needed (3 on the bottom, 1 on top).

2. High pressure for 6 minutes. Close and lock the lid and ensure the pressure valve is sealed, then select High Pressure and set the time for 6 minutes.
3. Pressure Release. Once the cook time is complete, quick release the pressure, being careful not to get your fingers or face near the steam release.
4. Once all the pressure has released, carefully unlock and remove the lid. Let cool for a few minutes before carefully lifting out the ramekins with oven mitts or tongs.
5. Let cool for at least 10 minutes before serving.

Nutrition

Calories: 129; Total fat: 1g; Protein: 3g; Sodium: 39mg; Fiber: 3g

Almond Balls

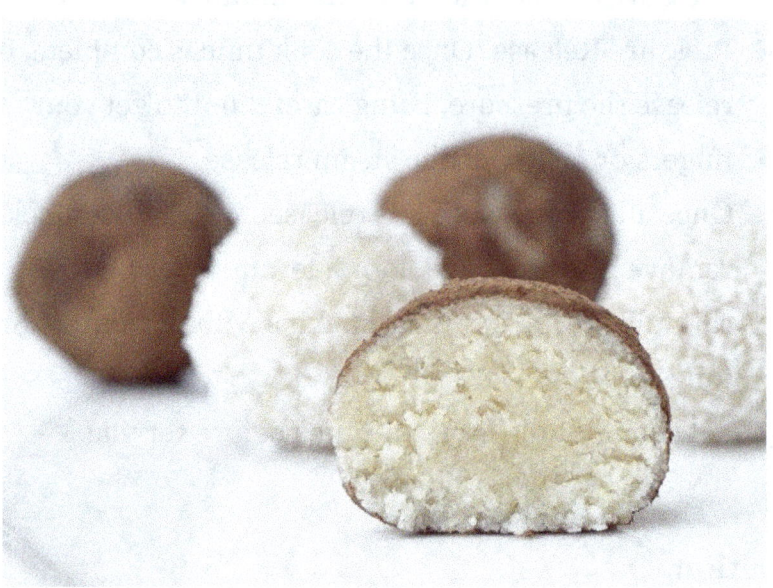

Preparation time: 10 minutes

Cooking time: 0 minutes

Servings: 6

Ingredients:
- ½ cup coconut oil, melted
- ¼ cup coconut flesh, unsweetened and shredded
- 5 tablespoons almonds, chopped
- 1 tablespoon stevia

Directions:

1. In a bowl, combine the coconut oil with the almonds and the other ingredients, stir well and spoon into round moulds.
2. Serve them cold.

Nutrition:

calories 194, fat 21.2, fiber 0.7, carbs 1, protein 1.4

Creamy Pineapple Mix

Preparation time: 10 minutes

Cooking time: 10 minutes

Servings: 4

Ingredients:

- 1 teaspoon nutmeg, ground
- 1 cup pineapple, peeled and cubed
- 1 teaspoon vanilla extract
- 1 cup coconut cream
- ½ cup stevia

Directions:

1. In a pan, combine the pineapple with the nutmeg and the other ingredients, toss, cook over medium heat for 10 minutes, divide into bowls and serve.

Nutrition:

calories 329, fat 32.7, fiber 0, carbs 2.5, protein 5.7

Cocoa Muffins

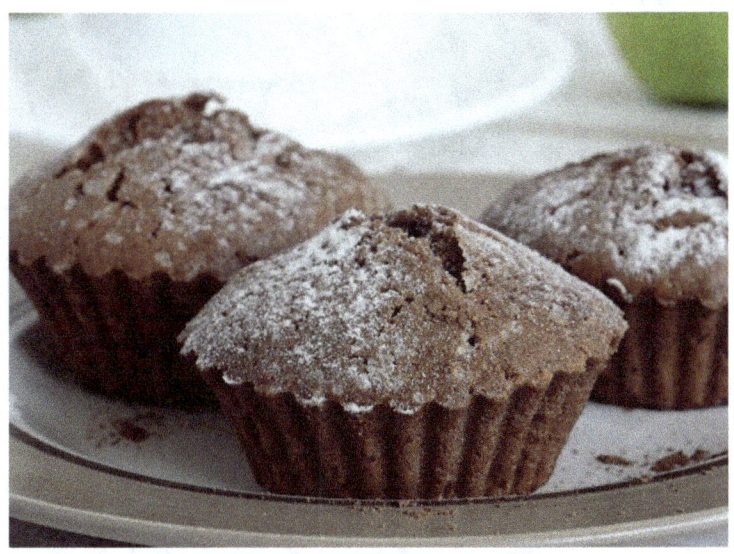

Preparation time: 10 minutes

Cooking time: 25 minutes

Servings: 6

Ingredients:

- ½ cup coconut oil, melted
- 3 tablespoons stevia
- ¼ cup cocoa powder
- 1 cup almond flour
- 3 tablespoons flaxseed mixed with 4 tablespoons water

- ¼ teaspoon vanilla extract
- 1 teaspoon baking powder
- Cooking spray

Directions:

1. In a bowl, combine the coconut oil with the stevia, the flour and the other ingredients except for the cooking spray and whisk well.
2. Grease a muffin pan with the cooking spray, divide the muffin mix in each mould, bake at 370 degrees F for 25 minutes, cool down and serve.

Nutrition:

calories 344, fat 35.1, fiber 3.4, carbs 8.3, protein 4.5

Chia and Strawberries Mix

Preparation time: 10 minutes

Cooking time: 0 minutes

Servings: 4

Ingredients:

- 1 cup strawberries, halved
- ¼ cup coconut milk
- 2 tablespoons chia seeds
- 1 tablespoon stevia

Directions:

1. In a bowl, combine the berries with the chia seeds, the milk and stevia and whisk well.
2. Divide the mix into bowls and serve cold.

Nutrition:

calories 265, fat 6.3, fiber 2, carbs 4, protein 6

Ginger Cream

Preparation time: 10 minutes

Cooking time: 10 minutes

Servings: 4

Ingredients:

- 2 tablespoons stevia
- 1 teaspoon vanilla extract
- 2 cups coconut cream
- 1 tablespoon cinnamon powder
- ¼ tablespoon ginger, grated
-

Directions:

1. In a pan, combine the cream with the stevia and other ingredients, stir, cook over medium heat for 10 minutes, divide into bowls and serve cold.

Nutrition:

calories 280, fat 28.6, fiber 2.7, carbs 7, protein 2.8

Coconut Chocolate Cake

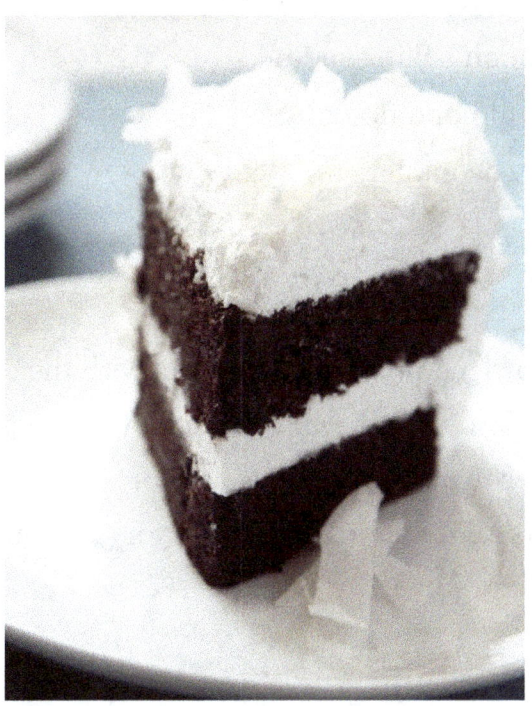

Preparation time: 10 minutes

Cooking time: 30 minutes

Servings: 12

Ingredients:

- 4 tablespoons flaxseed mixed with 5 tablespoons water
- 1 cup coconut flesh, unsweetened and shredded
- 1 teaspoon vanilla extract

- 4 tablespoons stevia
- 2 tablespoons lime zest
- 2 tablespoons cocoa powder
- 1 teaspoon baking soda
- 2 cups almond flour
- 2 cups coconut cream

Directions:

1. In a bowl, combine the flax meal with the coconut, the vanilla and the other ingredients, whisk well and transfer to a cake pan.
2. Cook the cake at 360 degrees F for 30 minutes, cool down and serve.

Nutrition:

calories 268, fat 23.9, fiber 5.1, carbs 9.4, protein 6.1

Lime Custard

Preparation time: 10 minutes

Cooking time: 20 minutes

Servings: 6

Ingredients:

- 1 pint almond milk
- 4 tablespoons lime zest, grated
- 3 tablespoons lime juice
- tablespoons stevia
- 3 tablespoons flaxseed mixed with 4 tablespoons water
- 2 teaspoons vanilla extract

Directions:

1. In a bowl, combine the almond milk with the lime zest, lime juice and the other ingredients, whisk well and divide into 4 ramekins.
2. Bake in the oven at 360 degrees F for 30 minutes.
3. Cool the custard down and serve.

Nutrition:

calories 234, fat 21.6, fiber 4.3, carbs 9, protein 3.5

Keto Flax Seed Waffles

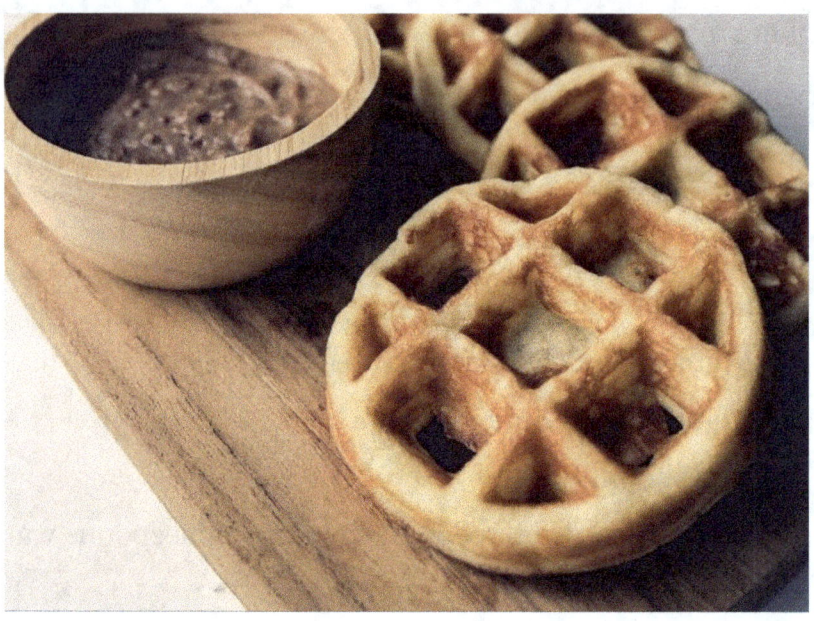

Preparation time: 20 minutes

Ingredients for 4 portions:

- 2 cups Golden Flax Seed
- 5 tbsp. Flax Seed Meal (mixed with 15 tbsp. Water)
- 1 tbsp. Baking Powder
- ⅓ cup Avocado Oil
- ½ cup Water

- 1 tsp. Sea Salt
- 1 tbsp. fresh Herbs (thyme, rosemary or parsley) or 2 tsp. cinnamon, ground

Directions:
1. Preheat the waffle-maker.
2. Combine the flax seed with baking powder with a pinch of salt in a bowl. Whisk the mixture.
3. Place the jelly-like flax seed mixture, some water and oil into the blender and pulse until foamy.
4. Transfer the liquid mixture to the bowl with the flax seed mixture. Stir until combined. The mixture must be fluffy.
5. Once it is combined, set aside for a couple of minutes. Add some fresh herbs or cinnamon. Divide the mixture into 4 servings.
6. Scoop each, one at a time, onto the waffle maker. Cook with the closed top until it's ready. Repeat with the remaining batter.
7. Eat immediately or keep in an air-tight container for a couple of weeks.

Cranberries and Avocado Pie

Preparation time: 10 minutes

Cooking time: 40 minutes

Servings: 4

Ingredients:

- 1 cup cranberries
- 1 cup avocado, peeled, pitted and mashed
- Cooking spray
- 1 cup coconut cream
- 1 cup stevia
- 1/3 cup almond flour
- 1 cup coconut, unsweetened and shredded
- ¼ cup avocado oil

Directions:

1. In a bowl, mix the cranberries with the avocado, the cream and the other ingredients except the cooking spray and whisk well.
2. Grease a cake pan with the cooking spray, pour the pie mix inside and bake at 350 degrees F for 40 minutes.
3. Cool the pie down, slice and serve.

Nutrition:

calories 172, fat 3.4, fiber 4.3, carbs 11.5, protein 4.5

Greek Chia Pudding (lacto)

Preparation Time: 20 minutes

Cooking Time: 0 minute

Servings: 3

Ingredients:

- 1 cup full-fat Greek yogurt
- ½ cup full-fat coconut milk
- 4-6 drops stevia sweetener (or alternatively, use low-carb maple syrup)
- ½ scoop organic soy protein powder (vanilla or chocolate flavor)
- 5 tbsp. chia seeds
- ¼ cup raspberries
- ¼ cup pecans (crushed)
- Optional: 1-2 tbsp. water

Directions:

1. In a medium-sized bowl, mix the yogurt with the coconut milk.
2. Stir in the protein powder and chia seeds until the protein powder is fully incorporated. Add some water if necessary.

3. Allow the pudding to sit for 2 minutes; then add the stevia sweetener and give the yogurt another stir.
4. Refrigerate the pudding overnight (or for at least 8 hours). This will guarantee a perfect pudding.
5. Top the pudding with the raspberries and crushed pecans; serve and enjoy!
6. Alternatively, store the pudding in an air-tight container and keep it in the fridge and consume within 4 days. Or, you can freeze the pudding for a maximum of 30 days and thaw at room temperature.

Nutrition:

Calories: 318kcal, Net Carbs: 6.5g, Fat: 26.6g, Protein: 11.9g, Fiber: 7.4g, Sugar: 4g

Nutty Protein Shake (vegan)

Preparation Time: 5 minutes

Cooking Time: 0 minute

Servings: 1

Ingredients:

- 2 tbsp. coconut oil
- 2 cups unsweetened almond milk
- 2 tbsp. peanut butter
- 1 scoop organic soy protein powder (chocolate flavor)
- 4-6 drops stevia sweetener
- 2-4 ice cubes
- Optional: 1 tsp. vegan creamer
- Optional: 1 tsp. cocoa powder

Directions:

1. Add all the above listed ingredients—except the optional ingredients—to a blender, and blend for 2 minutes.
2. Transfer the shake to a large cup or shaker. If desired, top the shake with the optional vegan creamer and/or cocoa powder.

3. Stir before serving, and enjoy!
4. Alternatively, store the smoothie in an air-tight container or a mason jar, keep it in the fridge, and consume within 3 days. Store for a maximum of 30 days in the freezer and thaw at room temperature.

Nutrition:

Calories: 618kcal, Net Carbs: 4.4g, Fat: 51.3g, Protein: 34g, Fiber: 4.9g, Sugar: 3g

Avocado Cucumber Soup

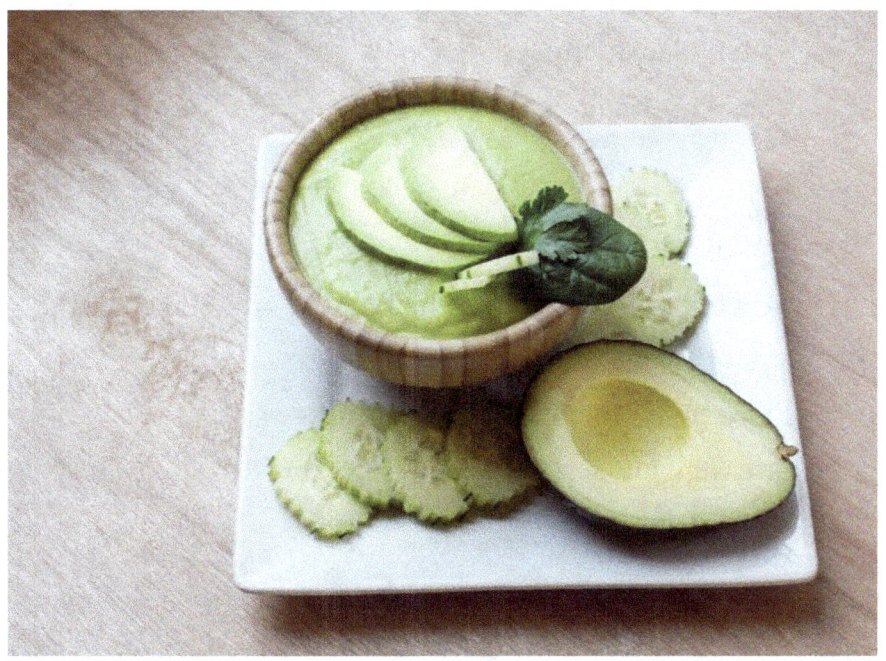

Preparation Time: 40 minutes

Cooking Time: 0 minute

Servings: 3

Ingredients:

- 1 large cucumber, peeled and sliced
- ¼ cup lemon juice
- ¾ cup water

- 2 avocados, pitted
- 2 garlic cloves
- 6 green onion
- ½ tsp black pepper
- ½ tsp pink salt

Directions:
1. Add all ingredients into the blender and blend until smooth and creamy.
2. Place in refrigerator for 30 minutes.
3. Stir well and serve chilled.

Nutrition:
Calories 73, Fat 3.7g, Carbohydrates 9.2g, Sugar 2.8g, Protein 2.2g, Cholesterol 0mg

NOTE

www.ingramcontent.com/pod-product-compliance
Lightning Source LLC
Chambersburg PA
CBHW070932080526
44589CB00013B/1489